SMART

PEPTIDES

**The Safe, Science-Based Way
to Build Muscle, Improve
Focus, Recover Faster, and
Biohack Your Way to Long-
Lasting Health**

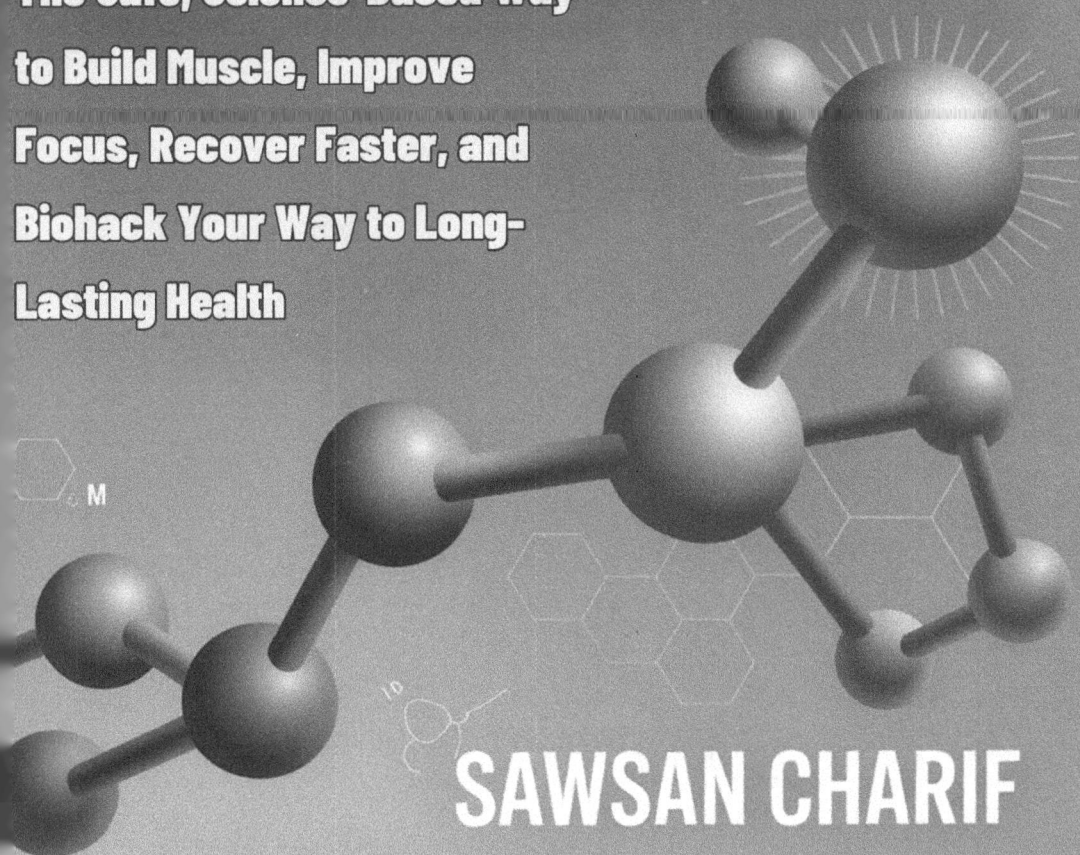

SAWSAN CHARIF

Smart Peptides

The Safe, Science-Based Way to Build Muscle, Improve Focus, Recover Faster, and Biohack your way to Long-Lasting Health

Sawsan Charif

BRAIN CORNER
PUBLISHING

Brain Corner Publishing

Contents

Disclaimer   VIII

Introduction   X
    What You'll Find in This Book
    Safety First, Always
    Your Journey Begins

1. The Peptide Foundation   1
    Science and Fundamentals
       The Building Blocks: Peptides Explained
       A Brief History of Peptides
       Myth vs. Reality: Peptides and Proteins
       Cell Talk: How Peptides Communicate in Your Body
       Beyond Basics: The Health Impact of Peptides
       Daily Life Enhancement: Practical Peptide Benefits
       Maximizing Impact: The Science of Bioavailability

2. Navigating the Peptide Landscape   11
    From Selection to Results
       Peptide Profiles: The Complete Guide
       Safety Shield: Critical Usage Guidelines
       Perfect Match: Aligning Peptides with Health Goals
       Legal and Ethical Compass: Navigating Responsibilities
       Administration Mastery: Methods and Techniques

Troubleshooting Toolkit: Solving Common Problems

3. Muscle Makers 22

Peptides for Strength and Recovery

Power Builders - Peptides That Pack a Punch

Recovery Accelerators: Healing Through Peptides

Admin Precision: Dosage and Timing for Muscle Enhancement

Success Stories: Real-World Muscle Transformations

4. Weight Management Masters 32

Peptides for Fat Loss

The Science of Peptides in Weight Management

GLP-1 Game-Changers: Revolutionary Weight Loss Peptides

Body Sculptors: Growth Hormone Secretagogues

Strategic Protocols: Weight Loss Peptide Programs

Lifestyle Integration: Maximizing Peptide Weight Loss

Transformation Stories: Weight Loss Success Through Peptides

5. Brain Boosters 44

Peptides for Cognitive Enhancement

Mind-Body Connection: How Peptides Enhance Brain Function

Mental Sharpeners: Focus and Memory Peptides

Calm Creator: Selank- The Anti-Anxiety Peptide

Focus Enhancer: Semax- The Cognitive Booster

Synergy Stacks: Combining Peptides with Nootropics

Mind Masters: Cognitive Enhancement Success Stories

6. Time Reversers 57

Peptides for Anti-Aging and Longevity

Youth Revolution: Peptides at the Anti-Aging Frontier

Skin Rejuvenator: GHK-Cu - The Copper Peptide

Life Extenders: Longevity Peptides Explained

Telomere Protector: Epitalon - The Longevity Peptide

Holistic Approach: Integrating Peptides with Longevity Practices

Risk-Benefit Balance: Safety in Anti-Aging Peptide Use

7. Skin Saviors   68

Skin Science: How Peptides Transform Your Complexion

Collagen Commanders: Peptides for Elasticity and Firmness

Product Navigator: Finding Effective Peptide Skincare

Skin Transformations: Real Results with Peptides

8. Athletic Edge   78

Peptides in Sports Performance

Performance Revolution: The Peptide Advantage in Sports

Endurance Enhancers: Peptides for Stamina and Performance

Supplement Showdown: Peptides vs. Traditional Options

Champion Profiles: Athletes' Experiences with Peptides

Ethical Playbook: Navigating Peptides in Competitive Sports

9. Healing Heroes   88

Peptides for Recovery and Repair

Tissue Mender: TB-500 and Thymosin Beta-4

Body Protector: BPC-157 - The Healing Compound

Immune Guardian: The Power of Thymosin Alpha-1

Inflammation Fighters: Peptide Solutions for Pain and Swelling

Recovery Chronicles: Real-Life Healing Stories

10. Mind Medicine   99

Peptides and Mental Health

Brain Chemistry: Peptides and Mental Wellness

Stress Soothers: Peptides for Calm and Balance

Mood Elevators: Peptides for Emotional Wellbeing

Mental Health Journeys: Transformative Peptide Stories

Integrative Approach: Mental Wellness Beyond Peptides

11. Wellness Integration   109

Creating Your Peptide Protocol

Personalized Planning: Creating Your Peptide Strategy

Nutritional Synergy: Peptides and Diet Working Together

Exercise Enhancement: Maximizing Workout Results with Peptides

Progress Tracking: Measuring Your Peptide Success

Mind-Body Balance: Mindfulness and Peptide Optimization

12. Safety Shield   119

Addressing Concerns and Misconceptions

Myth Busters: Debunking Common Peptide Misconceptions

Side Effect Spotlight: What to Watch For

Safety Protocols: Essential Guidelines for Protection

Special Considerations: Who Should Exercise Caution

Evidence-Based Confidence: Addressing Peptide Skepticism

13. Problem Solving   131

Troubleshooting Common Issues

Results Refinement: Managing Inconsistent Outcomes

Side Effect Solutions: Addressing Unexpected Reactions

Quality Control: Identifying and Avoiding Fake Products

Plateau Breakers: Overcoming Stalled Progress

Decision Guide: Problem-Solving Flowcharts

14. Future Horizons   141

Emerging Peptide Research

Research Frontiers: Breakthrough Peptide Discoveries

Precision Medicine: Personalized Peptide Therapies

Chronic Disease Management: Peptide Applications

Technology Accelerators: Tools Advancing Peptide Science

15. Practical Resources   152

Tools for Your Peptide Journey

Digital Trackers: Monitoring Your Peptide Progress

Integration Strategies

Choosing the Right Tools

Knowledge Sources: Finding Reliable Peptide Information

Community Connections: Building Your Peptide Support Network

Expert Perspectives: Insights from Peptide Pioneers

Next Steps: Continuing Your Peptide Education

16. Advanced Peptide Strategies   163

Cautions and Combinations

    The Fat-Killing Peptide That Went Too Far: A Cautionary Tale of Adipotide

17. Peptide Stacking Protocols   167

Peptide Stacking Made Simple: Protocols by Goal

Stack 1: Fat Loss & Metabolic Boost

Stack 2: Muscle Growth & Recovery

Stack 3: Focus, Mood & Mental Performance

Stack 4: Anti-Aging & Longevity

Stack 5: Gut Repair & Inflammation Control

Stack 6: Injury Recovery & Tissue Regeneration

Stacking Best Practices

Conclusion

What You've Accomplished

Key Takeaways for Practical Application

The Road Ahead

A Foundation for Future Exploration

Join Our Community

My Gratitude

Final Words of Inspiration

18. References   180

References

Disclaimer

—◄O►—

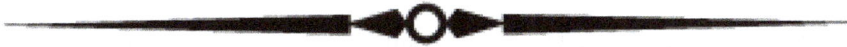

MEDICAL AND LEGAL DISCLAIMER
CRITICAL NOTICE: READ BEFORE PROCEEDING

Medical Disclaimer: This book is strictly for educational and informational purposes only. Nothing in this publication constitutes medical advice, diagnosis, or treatment recommendations. The information presented is for research and educational purposes only and should not be used to diagnose, treat, cure, or prevent any disease or medical condition.

Professional Medical Consultation Required: ALWAYS consult with a qualified healthcare provider before using any peptides or beginning any new health regimen. Individual responses to peptides vary significantly, and what may be safe for one person could be harmful to another based on medical history, current medications, and individual physiology.

FDA and Regulatory Status: Many peptides discussed in this book are not approved by the FDA for human consumption or therapeutic use. Some peptides exist in regulatory gray areas and their legal status may change. The purchase, possession, or use of certain peptides may be restricted or prohibited in your jurisdiction. for more context on evolving regulations, see [7].

Research vs. Therapeutic Use: All information is presented for research and educational purposes only. This book does not advocate for the illegal use of any substances. Readers are responsible for understanding and complying with all applicable laws and regulations in their jurisdiction.

No Medical Supervision: The author and publisher are not medical practitioners and do not provide medical supervision. Any use of peptides should be under the guidance of qualified healthcare professionals experienced in peptide therapy.

Liability Limitations: The author, publisher, distributors, and any associated parties expressly disclaim all liability for any adverse effects, injuries, or damages that may result from the use of information contained in this book. Use of this information is at your own risk.

Quality and Source Warnings: The book does not endorse any specific peptide suppliers or guarantee the quality, purity, or safety of any products. Counterfeit and contaminated peptides pose serious health risks.

Individual Responsibility: By reading this book, you acknowledge that:

- You are solely responsible for your health decisions

- You will seek professional medical advice before using any peptides

- You understand the legal and health risks involved

- You will comply with all applicable laws and regulations

Age Restriction: This information is intended for adults 18 years and older only.

Introduction

T he doctor's words hit me like a cold wave: "I want you to stand up and walk to the door and back."

"Why?" I asked, confused by such a simple request during what I thought was a routine checkup.

"I want to see if you can walk."

I was 65 years old, and in that moment, I realized my doctor was assessing me for frailty—treating me like I was already on the path to becoming a fragile, declining elderly person. Something inside me rebelled against that future. I wasn't ready to accept that aging meant inevitable weakness, dependence, or resignation to physical decline.

That day sparked a journey that would completely transform my understanding of what's possible as we age.

I'm not a medical professional or researcher. I'm someone who refused to accept that growing older meant growing weaker. What started as a personal quest to maintain my vitality and independence led me deep into the fascinating world of peptides—small chains of amino acids that promised a new frontier in building muscle, enhancing focus, accelerating recovery, and extending healthy lifespan.

Over the next several years, I immersed myself in research, consulted with experts, and carefully experimented with evidence-based approaches. The results have been remarkable: in less than a year of incorporating peptides into my wellness routine, I feel stronger, more energetic, and more vital than I have in decades. That doctor's walking test? I could probably run circles around his office now.

What You'll Find in This Book

This book isn't about miracle cures or fountain-of-youth fantasies. It's about the real, science-backed potential of peptides for people who want to take control of their aging process. Whether you're in your 40s looking to optimize performance, your 50s wanting to maintain strength and energy, or like me, determined to redefine what's possible in your 60s and beyond—this guide will show you how.

You'll discover:

- The real science behind how peptides work in your body

- Practical protocols for muscle building, weight management, and cognitive enhancement

- Safety guidelines and quality sourcing strategies

- Real-world success stories from people who've transformed their health

- Step-by-step guidance for creating your own personalized peptide strategy

Safety First, Always

Throughout this journey, I've learned that knowledge and caution must go hand in hand. This book emphasizes evidence-based approaches, professional guidance, and responsible use. Every recommendation is grounded in scientific research and real-world experience, with safety as the top priority.

Your Journey Begins

If you're reading this, you're probably facing your own moment of choice—will you accept conventional ideas about aging, or will you explore what's possible when science meets determination?

Let's rewrite the story of what it means to age well, one peptide at a time.

SPECIAL BONUS! THE PEPTIDE STARTER SAFETY KIT START YOUR JOURNEY RIGHT!

As a **small token of thanks for buying this book**, I am offering a free bonus gift to my readers.

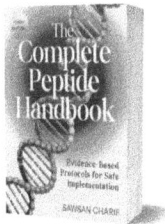

Starting peptides safely can make the difference between transformation and setbacks. Are you ready to begin your optimization journey with confidence, avoid costly mistakes, and maximize your results from day one?

In The Peptide Starter Safety Kit: Your Complete Guide to Safe Peptide Use for Beginners, I will share essential, actionable strategies to help you:

Source authentic peptides and avoid dangerous counterfeits

Create your personalized safety checklist before starting any protocol

Monitor progress effectively with tracking templates and biomarkers

Recognize warning signs and know when to adjust or seek help

Stack peptides safely with advanced combination guidelines

Whether you're a biohacker, athlete, health optimizer, or wellness enthusiast, this practical guide will ensure you start your peptide journey on solid ground.

BONUS: This safhttps://prod.content.atticus.io/images/175488yunNEy2wdh 3c_ce.pngety kit is your exclusive companion to the comprehensive Smart Peptides system—covering crucial details that could save you time, money, and health risks.

Start safe. Optimize smart. Transform with confidence.

Get FREE unlimited access to it and all of my new books by joining my Readers Club.

Chapter One

The Peptide Foundation

Science and Fundamentals

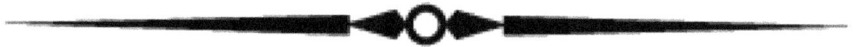

———————◆○◆———————

O ne evening, while sifting through a mountain of research papers, I stumbled upon an intriguing term: peptides. What seemed like a simple concept soon revealed a complex world of health possibilities. That spark of curiosity quickly turned into a deep passion.

Peptides—tiny chains of amino acids—stand at the frontier of modern health optimization. They serve as a bridge between cutting-edge science and personal wellness, offering promising benefits like enhanced strength, better sleep, accelerated recovery, and even longevity.

This chapter lays the groundwork for understanding peptide science, providing you with the foundation needed to explore these powerful molecules.

The Building Blocks: Peptides Explained

Peptides are both simple and sophisticated. At their core, they are short chains of amino acids linked by peptide bonds. They share the same building blocks as proteins, but are typically shorter—usually fewer than 50 amino acids in length [1]. This smaller size makes peptides less structurally complex than proteins, which often fold into intricate shapes to perform a wide array of biological functions.

Despite their simplicity, peptides are essential players in the body, acting as signaling molecules that transmit critical biological instructions.

Peptides can be classified in several ways depending on their function or origin:

Signaling peptides are crucial in cellular communication

Structural peptides help reinforce tissues and skin

Some peptides occur naturally in the body, while others are synthetically created in labs to enhance or mimic biological processes

A Brief History of Peptides

The story of peptides is a story of scientific evolution. Originally discovered in the early 20th century, peptides have since been the subject of groundbreaking research and innovation. Milestones like the discovery of insulin—a peptide hormone—laid the groundwork for therapeutic peptides used today [2].

From early experimentation to modern biohacking, peptides have transformed from obscure scientific curiosity into mainstream health tools with widespread applications.

Today, understanding peptides is vital for anyone interested in health optimization. They hold the potential to revolutionize wellness by offering targeted solutions for muscle growth, cognitive enhancement, and aging gracefully. As we explore this chapter, you'll gain a clearer picture of how peptides can play an integral part in your health strategy. With accurate information and practical insights, you'll be equipped to harness the power of peptides safely and effectively. Peptide therapy is gaining traction as a versatile, science-based strategy for improving physical, cognitive, and metabolic health . Peptides are often called the body's building blocks for good reason—they regulate essential physiological processes and adapt well to modern therapeutic strategies

Interactive Element: Reflection Exercise

Take a moment to reflect on what you hope to achieve with peptide use. Jot down three specific health goals where you think peptides could make an impact. Keep this list handy as we explore the possibilities in the chapters ahead.

Myth vs. Reality: Peptides and Proteins

Peptides and proteins often get mixed up in discussions about health and wellness. At their core, both are made of amino acids. Yet the number of these building blocks varies greatly between them.

Peptides are shorter, typically spanning 2 to 50 amino acids, while proteins are much longer and more complex, sometimes comprising hundreds or thousands of amino acids. This difference isn't just cosmetic—it's foundational. Proteins fold into intricate structures, essential for their diverse functions in the body. Peptides, smaller and simpler, don't require such elaborate folding. They remain more straightforward in structure, allowing them to act swiftly and effectively.

Functional Differences

Functionally, these molecules diverge significantly. Proteins serve as enzymes, catalyzing reactions crucial for life. They provide structural support, giving cells shape and integrity. Peptides, on the other hand, excel in communication. They act as signaling molecules, conveying messages between cells and triggering specific responses.

This distinction is crucial. For instance, peptides like insulin regulate blood sugar levels, while a protein like hemoglobin transports oxygen in the blood. Their roles underscore their unique contributions to our physiology.

Misunderstandings about peptides often arise from viewing them as merely smaller proteins. This oversimplification overlooks their unique therapeutic potentials. Peptides offer targeted interventions in health optimization. They're not just smaller proteins; they're specialized molecules with distinct roles. Therapeutic peptides have emerged as powerful tools in medicine, particularly in cancer treatments where their precision is invaluable.

Consider insulin—a peptide that has revolutionized diabetes management. Its small size allows it to efficiently regulate glucose levels. Compare this to hemoglobin, a protein responsible for oxygen transport. Hemoglobin's size and complexity are essential for its function but unnecessary for insulin's role. Similarly, therapeutic peptides target cancer cells with precision, unlike broader-spectrum treatments. These examples illustrate the distinct capabilities of peptides versus proteins.

Understanding these differences clarifies their applications and dispels common misconceptions. Recognizing peptides' unique strengths allows us to appreciate their role in health optimization and therapeutic interventions. This nuanced understanding empowers informed decisions, guiding us in leveraging peptides effectively for improved well-being.

Cell Talk: How Peptides Communicate in Your Body

Peptides act as the body's whisperers, relaying critical messages to maintain well-being. At the cellular level, their communication starts with receptor binding. Each peptide fits into its specific receptor like a key in a lock, initiating a conversation within the cell. This interaction triggers signal transduction pathways, a cascade of biochemical reactions that lead to a cellular response. Think of it as a relay race where the baton is passed from one runner to another, ensuring the message reaches its intended destination. This intricate process is what allows peptides to influence various bodily functions efficiently and specifically.

Examples in Action

Consider growth hormone-releasing peptides. These molecules stimulate the pituitary gland to release growth hormone, which then promotes tissue growth and repair. Such peptides play an instrumental role in muscle development and recovery, making them invaluable for athletes and fitness enthusiasts.

Another example is peptides involved in immune modulation. These peptides enhance immune responses, offering protection against infections and diseases. They fine-tune the immune system's activities, ensuring a balanced response to pathogens while minimizing the risk of autoimmune reactions.

Metabolic Influence

Peptides also wield influence over metabolic pathways. By regulating metabolism, they ensure that the body maintains adequate energy levels and efficient use of nutrients. Peptides that regulate glucose and lipid metabolism are crucial for maintaining energy balance, particularly in an era where metabolic disorders are prevalent. They help cells convert nutrients into usable energy, supporting overall vitality and endurance. This regulation is vital for those aiming to optimize their physical performance or manage weight effectively.

Homeostasis, the body's ability to maintain internal stability, heavily relies on peptides. These molecules participate in hormonal regulation, adjusting levels in response to changing conditions. During stress, for example, peptides modulate the stress response, preventing overreaction and maintaining equilibrium. Their role extends beyond immediate responses; they ensure long-term balance by constantly adjusting physiological processes. In essence, peptides are the body's diligent caretakers, tirelessly working behind the scenes to keep systems running smoothly and efficiently. Their impact is profound, foundational to our health and well-being, making them a vital focus for anyone seeking to biohack their body for lasting vitality.

Beyond Basics: The Health Impact of Peptides

Peptides extend their benefits far beyond basic biological functions, reaching into areas of health optimization that are both exciting and transformative.

Muscle and Skin Enhancement

One of their most celebrated roles is in muscle growth enhancement. Peptides like growth hormone secretagogues stimulate the release of growth hormone, which in turn supports muscle repair and development. This effect is invaluable for athletes striving for peak performance and individuals looking to maintain muscle mass as they age.

Additionally, peptides contribute significantly to skin health improvement. They enhance collagen production, which is crucial for maintaining skin elasticity and reducing signs of aging. This makes peptides a popular choice in skincare, offering a natural route to rejuvenation.

Cognitive Benefits

Cognitive enhancement is another realm where peptides shine. Certain peptides support neurotransmitter function, improving memory, focus, and overall mental clarity. This cognitive boost is particularly beneficial in our fast-paced world, where mental agility is as prized as physical strength.

Disease Prevention and Treatment

In disease prevention, peptides hold promising potential. Antimicrobial peptides, for instance, offer a natural defense against bacteria and viruses, reducing the risk of infections. In cancer therapy, specific peptides target cancer cells, minimizing damage to healthy tissue and enhancing treatment efficacy. These therapeutic applications highlight peptides' versatility in medical interventions.

Holistic Integration

Adopting a holistic approach with peptides involves integrating them into broader health strategies. When combined with proper nutrition and regular exercise, peptides amplify the benefits of a healthy lifestyle. They complement mental wellness practices as well. Peptides that influence neurotransmitters can enhance the effects of meditation and mindfulness, creating a balanced approach to well-being.

Real-world evidence supports these peptide benefits. Clinical trials have documented their effectiveness in various treatments, underscoring their role in modern medicine. For instance, antimicrobial peptides have shown success in treating resistant infections, while cancer therapies have leveraged peptide specificity for targeted action [2]. These examples illustrate the tangible impact peptides can have on health.

By incorporating peptides into daily routines, individuals can unlock a broader spectrum of health benefits. This integration is not just about addressing specific issues but about enhancing overall vitality. Peptides offer a unique opportunity to elevate personal wellness beyond conventional limits, paving the way for a healthier future.

Daily Life Enhancement: Practical Peptide Benefits

Peptides offer a multitude of enhancements that touch every corner of our health.

Physical Performance

For those striving for muscle growth and repair, peptides like growth hormone secretagogues stimulate muscle tissue regeneration, accelerating recovery post-exercise. It's akin to having a personal trainer inside your body, ensuring your muscles are nurtured and primed for action.

Cognitive function gets a noticeable boost from peptides, too. They fine-tune neurotransmitter systems, enhancing focus and elevating mood. Imagine sharpening your mind to a laser-like precision, ready to tackle any mental challenge with clarity and vigor.

Preventive Health

Peptides also hold a promising role in preventive health. They bolster the immune system, acting as vigilant sentinels that ward off intruders before they can cause harm. Anti-aging peptides rejuvenate skin by promoting collagen production, reducing wrinkles and ensuring your skin remains vibrant. These peptides offer more than cosmetic benefits; they support skin health at a cellular level, ensuring resilience against environmental stressors.

Real-World Success Story

Consider the story of a middle-aged office worker who incorporated peptides into her routine. She noticed enhanced energy levels and improved mood within weeks. Her skin appeared more youthful, and she experienced fewer colds throughout the year, attributing these changes to her peptide regimen. Documented clinical outcomes further support these benefits, with studies highlighting peptides' effectiveness in enhancing overall health markers.

Practical Integration

Incorporating peptides into daily life is practical and straightforward. Pairing them with a balanced diet and regular exercise amplifies their benefits. Monitoring and adjusting dosage based on personal responses can optimize results. Imagine starting your day with a peptide-enhanced smoothie, combining nutrition with cutting-edge science for maximum effect. This integration fosters a symbiotic relationship between lifestyle choices and peptide use, creating an environment where health flourishes.

Peptides are more than supplements; they are allies in the quest for optimal health. Mainstream health sources have begun emphasizing peptide therapy as a safe and accessible option for various conditions [61]. By understanding and utilizing them effectively, individuals can unlock new levels of vitality and longevity, making every day a step towards enhanced well-being.

Maximizing Impact: The Science of Bioavailability

Bioavailability is a term that sits at the heart of understanding peptide effectiveness. It refers to the proportion of a substance that enters the bloodstream and is available for use by the body. For peptides, high bioavailability means they can perform their intended functions more efficiently, whether it's building muscle or enhancing cognitive function. Several factors can affect this, including how peptides are absorbed and metabolized. A peptide's stability and the body's digestive enzymes can either enhance or hinder its absorption, impacting its therapeutic efficacy.

Delivery Methods Matter

Delivery methods play a crucial role in bioavailability:

- **Injectable peptides** often boast higher bioavailability because they bypass the digestive system, entering directly into the bloodstream where they can work quickly

- **Oral peptides**, while more convenient, face a gauntlet of digestive enzymes that can break them down before they reach circulation

- **Transdermal delivery systems**, like patches, offer a middle ground, slowly releasing peptides through the skin into the bloodstream over time

Factors Influencing Absorption

Several factors can influence bioavailability:

- **Peptide stability** is essential; unstable peptides degrade before their job begins

- The **digestive system's enzymatic activity** can also reduce effectiveness, breaking down peptides prematurely

- **Timing and dosage** are crucial for maximizing impact

Taking peptides on an empty stomach may enhance absorption for some types, while others benefit from being paired with specific nutrients or taken at particular times of day.

Optimization Strategies

Practical tips can help you maximize peptide bioavailability:

- Consider the **timing** of your dosage. Some peptides are best taken first thing in the morning or just before bed to align with natural hormone cycles

- **Synergistic supplements** such as certain vitamins and minerals can enhance absorption by creating a favorable environment for peptides to thrive

- Making small adjustments in how you consume peptides ensures you reap the full benefits they offer

As we explore these aspects, remember that understanding bioavailability isn't just for scientists. It's about empowering yourself to make informed decisions, ensuring your peptide use is as effective as possible. By considering these factors, you not only optimize your health but also make every effort count in your quest for vitality and well-being.

Chapter Two

Navigating the Peptide Landscape

From Selection to Results

———————◆O◆———————

Peptide Profiles: The Complete Guide

I magine discovering a toolbox filled with precision tools, each designed to upgrade a specific part of your body. That's exactly what peptides offer—a suite of specialized molecules tailored to optimize health and performance.

In this chapter, we'll explore the key peptides making waves in the wellness, recovery, and longevity communities.

BPC-157: The Healing Mechanic

BPC-157 is renowned for its ability to accelerate tissue repair and recovery. Think of it as a skilled mechanic fine-tuning your body's healing systems.

Synthesized from a natural protein found in gastric juice, BPC-157 promotes angiogenesis (the formation of new blood vessels) and enhances nitric oxide signaling.

These mechanisms make it especially effective for:

- Athletes recovering from injuries or surgery

- Individuals with chronic inflammation

- Muscle recovery and regeneration [5]

Bonus: It may also enhance growth hormone receptor activity in muscle tissue, contributing to strength and repair benefits.

Thymosin Beta-4: The Immune Conductor

Thymosin Beta-4 is your internal systems coordinator—like a conductor leading an orchestra of immune responses.

It plays a powerful role in:

- Wound healing

- Reducing inflammation

- Modulating immune function

This peptide doesn't just defend your body—it helps optimize recovery and regeneration, even offering cognitive benefits through improved neuroplasticity and reduced oxidative stress [6].

Melanotan

II: The Sunless Tan Enhancer

For those seeking a sun-kissed glow without harmful UV exposure, Melanotan II offers a fascinating option.

This peptide mimics the melanocyte-stimulating hormone (MSH), stimulating natural skin pigmentation. Beyond aesthetics, it may provide some protection from UV radiation damage.

How These Peptides Work

Each of these peptides operates through biochemical signaling:

- **BPC-157** binds to receptors that activate tissue repair pathways

- **Thymosin Beta-4** influences cell migration, gene expression, and immune balance

- **Melanotan II** activates melanocortin receptors to darken the skin naturally

Together, they represent just a slice of what targeted peptide therapy can do.

Mechanistically, each peptide operates at a biochemical level through receptor binding interactions. BPC-157 binds to specific receptors that modulate healing pathways, while Thymosin Beta-4 influences gene expression related to immune responses. These interactions are akin to unlocking doors within your cells, allowing peptides to perform their specialized functions.

Consider an athlete who incorporates BPC-157 into their recovery protocol after an intense training season. The peptide accelerates healing, allowing them to return to peak performance faster than expected. In an anti-aging clinic, Melanotan II is used to provide clients with a safe tanning solution as part of their skincare regimen. These scenarios highlight how peptides can be tailored to fit individual needs and goals.

Case Study: Athlete Recovery Protocol

An elite swimmer faced recurrent shoulder injuries due to intense training schedules. By incorporating BPC-157 into their regimen, they experienced reduced recovery time and enhanced muscle repair, leading to improved performance in subsequent competitions. This case illustrates the practical application and effectiveness of peptide therapies in real-world scenarios.

Safety Shield: Critical Usage Guidelines

When using peptides, safety takes center stage. Keep them cool and dry, like a precious artifact, because improper storage can degrade their effectiveness. Reliable suppliers are crucial. Vet them as you would a new doctor—trustworthy and backed by solid credentials. This ensures you get what you expect, free from contaminants that could harm.

Understanding Side Effects

Be aware of potential side effects. Common issues can include:

- Injection site reactions, akin to a small bee sting

- Hormonal imbalances that may disrupt your body's rhythm

Stay vigilant and manage these by monitoring your body's responses closely. Adjustments can include changing injection spots or altering dosage under guidance.

Dosage Considerations

Speaking of dosages, these aren't just arbitrary numbers. They should align with your health objectives, whether it's muscle gain or cognitive enhancement. Start with the lowest effective dose and increase cautiously. Self-administration requires careful technique. Subcutaneous injections are common, needing precision and cleanliness to avoid complications.

Professional Guidance

Don't go it alone; a healthcare professional is an invaluable ally. They bring expertise to your peptide regimen, providing insights and adjustments you might miss. Regular check-ups ensure you're on the right path and help catch any issues before they spiral. Think of this as having a co-pilot to navigate the often complex landscape of peptide use.

In essence, managing peptides is about creating a robust framework to support their benefits. By prioritizing safety protocols and professional advice, you set the stage for a successful experience. This approach not only protects your health but maximizes the positive impacts peptides can have on your life.

Perfect Match: Aligning Peptides with Health Goals

Understanding your health goals is the first step in choosing the right peptides. Do you aim for fat loss or metabolic enhancement? Perhaps improved sleep quality and recovery are your priorities. Defining these objectives helps you select peptides that align with your specific needs.

Peptide Selection Examples

For instance, if you're focused on growth hormone release, CJC-1295 might be your go-to. It's known for stimulating hormone secretion, which supports muscle growth and fat metabolism. If appetite control and weight management are on your radar, consider Ipamorelin. This peptide helps regulate hunger levels and aids in weight management by mimicking ghrelin, a hunger hormone.

Customization Strategy

Once you've identified your goals, it's time to match them with the right peptides. Think of this as creating a customized approach where each peptide serves a specific purpose in your health optimization plan. Customization plays a big role here. Adjusting dosages based on how your body responds is crucial. Some people might need higher doses, while others achieve results with less. It's all about finding what works for you. Sometimes combining peptides can amplify effects, creating a synergy that enhances overall benefits.

Important Considerations

But it's not just about picking the right peptides and dosages; you must also be aware of potential contraindications. Pre-existing health conditions or interactions with current medications can influence your peptide selection. Always consider these factors to avoid undesirable effects. A healthcare provider can guide you through this process, ensuring your safety.

Personalizing your peptide protocol involves trial and error, patience, and listening to your body. Remember, what works for one person might not work for another. Keep track of your progress and be open to adjustments. By aligning peptides with your health goals and customizing their use, you set the stage for achieving desired outcomes effectively and safely. This approach not only maximizes benefits but also minimizes risks, allowing you to biohack your way to improved health and wellness.

Legal and Ethical Compass: Navigating Responsibilities

Understanding the Legal Landscape

Understanding the legal landscape of peptides is crucial. In the U.S., the FDA categorizes peptides as drugs rather than supplements if they have therapeutic claims, which means they must meet stringent approval processes. However, the regulatory environment isn't uniform worldwide. In Europe, regulations vary significantly across countries, with some treating peptides under medical product legislation, while others view them as supplements. This patchwork of rules makes it imperative for you to stay informed about the specific legal status in your region. What's accepted in one place might be restricted in another.

Ethical Considerations

Ethical considerations are just as important. The use of peptides in competitive sports raises significant concerns about fairness and integrity. Anti-doping agencies closely monitor peptide use, and athletes found using banned substances face severe consequences. Beyond sports, the sourcing of peptide materials poses ethical questions. Are the peptides produced sustainably? Are they tested ethically? These are questions worth asking to ensure that your health choices align with your values.

Staying Compliant

To navigate these complexities, staying informed is key. Regularly check for updates from regulatory bodies like the FDA or international equivalents to ensure compliance. Transparency with healthcare providers is crucial too. Discussing your peptide use openly helps them guide you safely and legally, providing a safety net for your health journey.

Ethics play a vital role in personal peptide use as well. Balancing personal goals with ethical responsibilities means considering not just the benefits to yourself but the broader implications of your actions. Engaging in informed and responsible use involves understanding both the potential impacts on your body and the ethical landscape surrounding peptides. This approach ensures that your pursuit of health and vitality doesn't come at a cost to integrity or fairness.

By keeping these legal and ethical dimensions in mind, you make informed choices that protect your health and well-being while respecting broader societal norms. This balance is crucial, ensuring that your path to enhanced wellness is both safe and responsible.

Administration Mastery: Methods and Techniques

Delivery Methods

Choosing the right method to administer peptides can hugely impact their effectiveness.

Subcutaneous Injections: Delivered just under the skin, these are popular for their direct absorption. They're like sending a direct message to your body, ensuring the peptide gets where it needs to go without much delay.

Intramuscular Injections: Offer faster absorption and are suited for larger doses, making them ideal for those needing a quick response.

Oral Administration: While convenient, this is limited to peptides stable enough to withstand digestive processes—a feat not all peptides can achieve.

Topical Applications: Perfect for skin-targeted peptides like those enhancing dermal health.

The choice of route depends on several factors, including bioavailability, user comfort, and the specific peptide's purpose. For instance, while subcutaneous injections might work best for ease and simplicity, someone prioritizing rapid effects might lean towards intramuscular options.

Best Practices for Self-Administration

Comparative studies show varying efficacy among these routes. Subcutaneous injections often reign supreme in terms of reliable absorption, while oral peptides like desmopressin provide a convenient alternative where stability allows. When administering peptides yourself, maintaining proper technique is crucial:

- Clean your hands and the injection site thoroughly

- Use fresh needles and syringes to avoid contamination and infection

- Rotate injection sites to prevent irritation and tissue damage

- The upper thigh or abdomen are common sites for subcutaneous injections

- Ensure you have all necessary tools like alcohol swabs and a safe disposal container

Dosage Guidelines

Dosage isn't a one-size-fits-all scenario either. It hinges on factors like your weight, age, and overall health status. Start with the minimal effective dose to gauge your body's reaction. IGF-1 LR3, for example, typically follows a weekly dosage protocol, while CJC-1295 involves specific cycles and frequencies. Adjustments should be based on individual responses, monitoring for signs of under or overdosing. Regular health checkups and lab tests can guide these adjustments, ensuring safety and efficacy. Cycling and stacking peptides can prevent tolerance development and enhance effects by using complementary peptides strategically. This approach helps maximize benefits while minimizing potential downsides, keeping your peptide regimen both effective and safe.

Troubleshooting Toolkit: Solving Common Problems

Common Challenges

Navigating the peptide landscape isn't always smooth sailing. You might encounter issues like ineffective results or unexpected side effects. These hiccups can be frustrating, leaving you questioning your regimen. But fear not—these challenges are part of the process and often have simple solutions. When results don't match expectations, it could be a matter of dosage or the administration route. A small adjustment can make a world of difference. Ensure your peptides are stored correctly and sourced from reputable suppliers to maintain their efficacy.

When to Seek Help

Sometimes, the body reacts unpredictably, leading to adverse effects. Mild reactions can often be managed at home, but some situations require professional intervention. Persistent adverse effects or lack of improvement despite adjustments are signals to consult a healthcare provider. They can offer insights and potentially recommend alternative strategies.

Prevention Strategies

Preventing future issues involves keeping detailed logs of your usage and responses. These logs can act as a guide, helping you spot patterns and make necessary tweaks. Regular consultations with a peptide-savvy healthcare professional are invaluable. They provide an external perspective and ensure you're on the right track.

Systematic Approach

When dealing with peptide-related problems, a systematic approach like a troubleshooting decision tree can be incredibly helpful:

1. Start with assessing symptoms progressively

2. Identify potential causes

3. Make necessary adjustments in administration technique or dosage

4. If minor side effects occur, simple management techniques often suffice

5. For serious adverse reactions, immediate action and professional consultation are crucial

Following best practices in storage and handling, alongside quality verification procedures, can prevent many issues from arising in the first place.

As you navigate this complex yet rewarding world of peptides, remember that troubleshooting is part of the journey. Don't hesitate to seek help when needed—it's a sign of strength and dedication to your health goals. Embrace these challenges as opportunities for growth and learning.

As we wrap up this chapter on practical peptide use, it's clear that facing challenges head-on equips you with the knowledge to optimize your health journey effectively. With the right tools and mindset, you're well-prepared to tackle any obstacles on the path to vitality. Moving forward, we'll explore even more advanced strategies to amplify your peptide experience in the next chapter.

Chapter Three

Muscle Makers

Peptides for Strength and Recovery

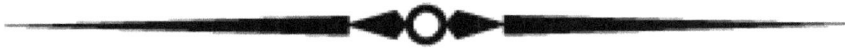

—————————◀O▶—————————

Power Builders—Peptides That Pack a Punch

Picture yourself in the gym—surrounded by the clanking of weights, the hum of focus, and that familiar mix of sweat and determination in the air. You're not just lifting for strength; you're sculpting a better version of yourself. And behind the scenes, peptides like IGF-1 LR3 and Follistatin work as powerful allies in that transformation. They're not just about raw power; they transform how your muscles grow and recover.

IGF-1 LR3: The Growth Catalyst

IGF-1 LR3 is a muscle-building powerhouse. It stimulates protein synthesis within cells and promotes muscle hypertrophy—the actual growth of muscle fibers.

Think of IGF-1 LR3 as flipping the switch on your body's internal construction crew:

- Faster recovery

- Enhanced growth signals

- Greater strength potential

By mimicking insulin-like growth factors naturally found in the body, it encourages lean muscle mass while supporting fat metabolism and cellular repair. This peptide essentially turns on the body's muscle-building machinery, helping you gain strength more efficiently [11].

Follistatin: The Muscle Growth Unleasher

Follistatin takes a different path to growth. It inhibits myostatin, a protein that limits muscle growth. Imagine removing the safety cap on a high-performance engine—Follistatin removes the biological brake that keeps your muscle size in check.

By suppressing myostatin:

- Muscle growth can exceed normal limits

- Gains are more noticeable

- Training outcomes can be amplified significantly

Follistatin works by activating satellite cells—those dormant helpers on the surface of muscle fibers. These cells multiply and fuse with existing fibers, increasing both their size and strength. It's like laying extra bricks to make a wall thicker and stronger [12].

How These Peptides Work

These peptides work by activating satellite cells—dormant cells that reside on the surface of muscle fibers. Once activated, these cells multiply and integrate with existing muscle fibers, increasing their size and potency. The process is akin to adding new bricks to a building, fortifying its structure. Enhanced protein synthesis follows, ensuring that your body has the necessary resources to repair and build muscle tissues post-exercise.

Who Benefits?

These peptides are ideal for:

- Athletes seeking performance gains

- Bodybuilders pushing for the next level of size

- Rehabilitation patients needing rapid muscle repair

While powerful, they're not a shortcut—they're a scientific enhancement to an already solid training foundation.

Important Considerations

However, it's important to be aware of potential hurdles when using muscle-building peptides. While they offer significant benefits, there's a risk of unnatural muscle growth if not used judiciously [13]. Balancing peptide use with natural training is crucial. Your body needs time to adapt to changes in muscle mass; rushing can lead to injury or imbalances.

Interactive Element: Muscle Growth Tracker

Consider starting a muscle growth tracker in your fitness journal. Record your workouts, peptide intake, and any changes in muscle size or strength. This practice not only helps in monitoring progress but also provides insight into how well your current regimen is working.

Incorporating peptides into your routine requires thoughtful planning and expert guidance. Consulting with healthcare professionals ensures that you're using these powerful substances safely and effectively. By understanding their mechanisms and potential benefits, you position yourself to unlock new levels of strength and recovery.

Recovery Accelerators: Healing Through Peptides

Imagine finishing a grueling workout and waking up the next day without that familiar soreness. It's not magic, but rather the power of peptides like BPC-157 and Thymosin Beta-4 (TB-4).

BPC-157: The Tissue Healer

BPC-157 works wonders for tissue healing. It operates by promoting angiogenesis, which is the formation of new blood vessels. This process enhances blood flow to damaged areas, accelerating recovery. Think of it as a natural repair kit for your body, mending tissues and reducing inflammation in ways traditional methods might overlook.

TB-4: The Regeneration Specialist

TB-4, on the other hand, excels in tissue regeneration. It reduces fibrosis—the thickening and scarring of connective tissue—which can otherwise slow recovery. By facilitating cell migration and modulating inflammation, TB-4 ensures that your body heals efficiently and effectively.

Dosing Protocols

When it comes to dosing, precision is key. For IGF-1 LR3, a common recommendation is a weekly dosage, allowing your body to integrate it gradually without overwhelming your system. CJC-1295 often follows a different protocol with cyclical dosing, promoting sustained release and effectiveness over time. These peptides require careful consideration of timing and quantity to maximize their benefits.

Cellular Recovery Mechanisms

At the cellular level, the recovery mechanisms of these peptides are fascinating. They enhance blood flow to muscles, ensuring that essential nutrients and oxygen reach the tissues that need them most. This increased circulation not only speeds up recovery but also reduces oxidative stress—a harmful process that can damage cells after intense exercise. Peptides also play a pivotal role in cell migration pathways, guiding cells to where they're needed most for effective tissue repair.

Integration with Traditional Recovery

Integrating peptides with traditional recovery strategies can amplify results. Physical therapy benefits from the accelerated healing peptides provide, making sessions more effective and shortening recovery timelines. Proper nutrition complements peptide use by supplying the building blocks necessary for muscle repair. Together, these elements create a robust recovery protocol that supports overall wellness.

Scientific Evidence

Scientific studies back these claims with compelling evidence. Clinical trials have shown significant improvements in recovery times for athletes using these peptides[14]. Peer-reviewed studies in sports medicine further validate their efficacy [15], providing a solid foundation for their use in recovery protocols. This research not only highlights the potential of peptides but also assures users of their safety and effectiveness when used correctly.

Incorporating peptides into your recovery regimen can be transformative, offering benefits that extend beyond muscle repair. It's about optimizing how your body heals and improving overall resilience. By understanding these mechanisms and utilizing them effectively, you can enhance your recovery process, allowing you to push your limits while maintaining optimal health and wellness.

Admin Precision: Dosage and Timing for Muscle Enhancement

Starting Smart with Dosing

When it comes to dosing peptides for muscle building and recovery, precision is your best friend and ally in achieving your fitness goals. Initial dosing protocols set the stage for how your body will react, providing a framework upon which effective muscle enhancement strategies can be developed.

Start with the lowest effective dose; this cannot be overstated, as gauging your body's response at this preliminary stage lays the groundwork for successful peptide therapy. This cautious approach is not only about preventing undue harm but also allows you a unique opportunity to observe how your body reacts to these powerful agents. After establishing a baseline with this gentle introduction, you can carefully consider any potential adjustments based on your individual physiological response.

Some may find they need slightly more to see desired and observable results in muscle size and recovery, while others may find that a conservative dose is sufficient. The key is to consistently monitor, evaluate the outcomes, and make adjustments as biocompatibility warrants.

Timing for Maximum Impact

Timing is another critical element in maximizing peptide efficacy and can make a substantial difference in the benefits you can reap. Administering peptides at the right moment, strategically planned around your workouts, can significantly enhance their effectiveness and optimize muscle building.

Pre-workout injections

might give you an edge by priming your muscles, ensuring they are biochemically ready for the upcoming exertions. The biochemical support provided allows muscles to work under optimal conditions, enhancing performance and boosting energy levels during the most demanding physical activities.

Post-exercise timing

pivots towards accelerating recovery. Injecting peptides after a workout supports a more efficient muscle repair process, decreasing downtime between sessions and allowing for significantly more consistent progress towards your goals.

Common Mistakes to Avoid

However, it's important to acknowledge that common mistakes can derail even the most well-intentioned peptide plans:

- **Overdosing** is one frequent error that must be avoided; it can lead to unwanted side effects, such as hormonal imbalances or even negating the benefits of peptides by overwhelming your body's systems

- **Misalignment** in timing and dosage can lead to missed opportunities for peak benefits or, worse, potential injuries that set back progress

- It's crucial to align your peptide use with your overall exercise routines, ensuring that your regimen is not only effective but also safe

Long-term Effectiveness Strategies

To maintain peptide effectiveness over time and ensure continued responsiveness, consider cycling them as part of your strategy. This approach prevents the dreaded onset of desensitization, a state where the body becomes accustomed to a constant influx of peptides and stops responding as effectively.

Cycling typically involves taking deliberate breaks from peptide use, or alternating with different peptides, which helps keep your body's receptors responsive and engaged. Additionally, combining peptides with supportive supplements such as amino acids or creatine can innovate and amplify their benefits. These supplements provide the necessary raw materials that your body needs to maximize peptide efficacy, offering a holistic approach to muscle enhancement.

Peptide use demands a thoughtful and well-considered approach, one that balances the science of supplementation with personal observation and experience. By understanding and adhering to initial dosing protocols, and making informed, thoughtful adjustments, you create a responsive and individualized plan that aligns seamlessly with your unique physiological makeup. Proper timing, carefully synchronized with your workouts, enhances the synergistic effect between peptides and physical exertion, maximizing your gains while minimizing the necessary recovery time between sessions.

Success Stories: Real-World Muscle Transformations

Peptides have quietly revolutionized how athletes and bodybuilders achieve their muscle goals. Their stories, rich in diversity and outcome, showcase the transformative potential of these small chains of amino acids.

The Elite Sprinter

Take, for instance, an elite sprinter who turned to peptides to boost explosive power. Through the strategic use of specific peptides, their sprinting times improved remarkably, allowing them to shave precious seconds off their personal bests. This isn't just about raw speed; it's about harnessing the body's biochemistry to achieve a level of performance once thought unreachable. The sprinter's experience underscores how peptides can refine and enhance the body's natural capabilities.

The Endurance Athlete

On a different spectrum, consider the endurance athlete who used peptides to maintain stamina during grueling long-distance runs. Peptides supported muscle endurance and delayed fatigue, essential for pushing through those final miles when every step feels like a mountain. Their testimony speaks volumes about how these compounds can be tailored to suit diverse athletic needs, from short bursts of power to sustained energy over time.

The Bodybuilder's Transformation

Then there's the bodybuilder whose transformation is nothing short of spectacular. With a carefully curated peptide protocol designed to maximize muscle gains while ensuring proper recovery, they achieved a physique that was not just about size but symmetry and proportion. Their journey highlights the importance of precision in peptide use, tailoring each dose and timing it perfectly with training cycles for optimal results.

Key Lessons Learned

Lessons from these stories are invaluable:

- **Personalized protocols** emerge as a key takeaway—what works for one might not work for another

- **Individual responses** to peptides can vary, making it crucial to adapt usage based on specific goals and physiological needs

- **Professional guidance** plays a pivotal role here. Having an expert to fine-tune your regimen can mean the difference between success and setbacks

Experts help navigate potential pitfalls, ensuring safe and effective use of peptides in your quest for muscle optimization.

Visual Evidence of Progress

Visual elements can add another layer of engagement, offering tangible evidence of progress. Imagine graphs that chart muscle gain over time or infographics that distill complex peptide benefits into digestible insights. These tools not only inspire but educate, providing a visual roadmap of what's possible with peptide use.

These stories weave a tapestry of success, illustrating the myriad ways peptides can be applied to achieve different muscle-related objectives. They aren't just tales of triumph; they're blueprints for what's achievable with the right approach and mindset. They emphasize that while peptides are powerful tools, their real strength lies in how they're used—strategically, thoughtfully, and under expert guidance.

As we conclude this chapter on muscle transformations through peptides, remember that these success stories are as much about the journey as the destination. Each one offers a unique perspective on how to integrate peptides into your fitness regimen effectively and safely. Moving forward, we'll explore how these strategies can be applied to enhance your overall health and recovery in our next chapter on optimizing sleep and longevity.

Chapter Four

Weight Management Masters

Peptides for Fat Loss

———————◆O◆———————

The Science of Peptides in Weight Management

I magine standing in front of your mirror, feeling the weight of yesterday's choices. Now picture a tool that could help guide those choices toward a healthier you. Peptides are that tool, working at a cellular level to help regulate weight, appetite, and metabolism.

Appetite Regulation Through Hormonal Signals

Peptides influence weight primarily by modulating hormones like leptin and ghrelin, which control hunger and satiety.

- **Leptin** signals fullness to the brain, reducing snacking and late-night cravings

- **Ghrelin** triggers hunger, and certain peptides suppress its activity, helping you feel satisfied longer

This natural hormone signaling makes smaller meals feel more filling—without relying on willpower alone.

Fat Burning & Metabolism Enhancement

Peptides also activate lipolysis, the process that breaks down stored body fat into usable energy. By unlocking fat from storage, they make it easier for your body to burn fat even at rest.

In addition:

- They increase metabolic rate, which means you burn more calories—even while sleeping or sitting

- Some improve insulin sensitivity, enhancing glucose management and reducing fat accumulation around the midsection

The Gut-Brain Connection

Peptides also affect the gut-brain axis, a powerful communication channel between your digestive and nervous systems. They modulate activity in the hypothalamus, the part of the brain that regulates hunger, so you're eating out of need—not habit.

By shifting internal signals, peptides help:

- Reduce cravings

- Improve meal timing

- Prevent binge-eating patterns

Diverse peptides tackle weight through different pathways. Some focus on direct fat mobilization, while others regulate appetite via the central nervous system. There are also peptides that enhance insulin sensitivity. This improvement aids in better glucose management and reduces fat accumulation, offering an additional layer of weight control.

Backed by Science

These effects aren't theoretical. Clinical studies have consistently demonstrated the impact of peptides like GLP-1 agonists, AOD-9604, and Tesamorelin on:

- Fat reduction

- Visceral weight loss

- Appetite suppression

- Improved metabolic function [16]

Interactive Element: Reflection Exercise

Consider writing down your current habits related to eating and exercise. Reflect on how incorporating peptides could influence these habits positively. This exercise not only clarifies your expectations but also helps in setting realistic goals for your weight management journey.

Peptides offer a potent strategy for those seeking to manage their weight effectively. Understanding their mechanisms helps harness their full potential in achieving your health goals.

GLP-1 Game-Changers: Revolutionary Weight Loss Peptides

Semaglutide: The Appetite Controller

Semaglutide represents a remarkable leap in weight management. It works by mimicking the effects of GLP-1, a hormone that enhances insulin secretion. This hormone plays a crucial role in regulating blood sugar levels and controlling appetite. By slowing gastric emptying, it prolongs the sensation of fullness after meals, reducing overall calorie intake. According to experts, Semaglutide remains one of the most effective peptides for sustainable weight loss [17].

Dosage protocols involve a gradual increase over weeks to minimize side effects and allow the body to adapt. Expected outcomes include significant weight loss within a few months, with clinical data showing impressive reductions in body weight (Medical News Today, n.d.).

Tirzepatide: The Dual-Action Powerhouse

Tirzepatide stands out with its dual-action approach, targeting both GLP-1 and GIP receptors. This dual mechanism amplifies its efficacy, offering enhanced results over single-mechanism peptides. By activating these pathways, Tirzepatide bolsters insulin sensitivity and curbs appetite, leading to more pronounced fat loss. It's particularly beneficial for individuals struggling with both insulin resistance and excess weight. However, it's essential to consider contraindications such as severe gastrointestinal disorders when contemplating its use. Detailed pharmacological profiles confirm Tirzepatide's dual action as both a GLP-1 and GIP receptor agonist [18].

Retatrutide: The Triple-Action Innovation

Retatrutide is at the forefront of peptide innovation, acting as a triple agonist by targeting GLP-1, GIP, and glucagon receptors simultaneously. This multifaceted approach not only aids in weight reduction but also enhances overall metabolic health. While still under investigation, early research suggests potential benefits far beyond traditional weight loss solutions, making it a promising candidate for future therapies.

Comparing the Options

When comparing these peptides, efficacy and side effect profiles vary. Clinical studies reveal substantial weight loss percentages with all three peptides, but their side effects differ in incidence and severity. One study found that GLP-1 receptor agonists led to measurable improvements in cardiovascular risk factors alongside weight loss [19]. Semaglutide users report mild gastrointestinal discomfort, whereas Tirzepatide's dual action may lead to more pronounced changes in glucose metabolism. Retatrutide's triple targeting introduces complexities yet to be fully understood but promises broader health benefits. Cost-benefit considerations are crucial; while these peptides offer impressive results, their financial implications must be weighed carefully against potential health gains.

Peptide	Mechanism	Benefits	Drawbacks	Ideal For
Semaglutide	GLP-1 agonist (Appetite control, insulin release)	Reduces appetite, effective weight loss, promotes satiety	GI discomfort, slow dosage titration	Appetite control, moderate sustainable loss
Tirzepatide	Dual GLP-1 & GIP agonist (Improved insulin sensitivity & fat loss)	Enhanced weight loss, better insulin response	Stronger glucose shifts, not for GI issues	Insulin resistance + fat loss combo
Retatrutide	Triple GLP-1, GIP & Glucagon agonist (Metabolic boost + weight loss)	Broad metabolic gains, promising early data	Still experimental, unknown risks	Advanced biohackers, metabolic optimization

Body Sculptors: Growth Hormone Secretagogues

Ipamorelin: The Fat Targeting Specialist

Imagine targeting that stubborn belly fat with precision. Ipamorelin, a growth hormone secretagogue, offers a unique edge by specifically mobilizing visceral adipose tissue. It works by stimulating growth hormone release, which in turn triggers the breakdown of fat stores, particularly around the abdomen. This targeted action is like having a laser-focused approach to fat loss, ensuring that you're chiseling away at the areas that matter most.

What sets Ipamorelin apart is its ability to preserve lean body mass while promoting fat reduction, making it a favorite for those who want to trim down without sacrificing muscle tone. Its effects are further amplified when combined with a consistent exercise routine, creating a synergistic impact on body composition.

CJC-1295 and Ipamorelin: The Dynamic Duo

When exploring combinations like CJC-1295 and Ipamorelin, the benefits multiply. These two peptides work in harmony, each enhancing the other's effects. CJC-1295 extends the half-life of growth hormone release, creating a sustained effect that complements Ipamorelin's sharp, short bursts. By optimizing dosing schedules—often using CJC-1295 as a baseline with periodic Ipamorelin injections—users can experience a powerful growth hormone pulse that supports both fat loss and muscle gain. Clinical use cases highlight this duo's effectiveness for fat reduction and anti-aging [20]. This combination isn't just about losing fat; it's about sculpting your body with precision.

GHRP-2 vs. GHRP-6: Appetite Considerations

GHRP-2 and GHRP-6 also deserve attention for their roles in body composition. While both stimulate growth hormone release, they differ in hunger modulation. GHRP-6 increases appetite, making it ideal for individuals looking to bulk up, whereas GHRP-2 is more neutral, providing growth hormone benefits without significant hunger changes. This distinction allows for tailored approaches depending on whether your goal is to gain mass or maintain a lean physique. Their potency in stimulating growth hormone makes them effective tools for enhancing muscle growth and fat loss.

Preserving Muscle During Fat Loss

In periods of caloric restriction, maintaining muscle mass becomes crucial. Peptides like these offer anti-catabolic benefits, supporting protein synthesis and reducing muscle breakdown. They not only help ensure that your hard-earned muscle is preserved during weight loss but also enhance recovery post-workout. By supporting lean tissue retention, these peptides provide a safety net against muscle loss, allowing you to focus on shedding fat without compromising strength or performance.

Peptide	Key Function	Best For	Unique Feature	Drawbacks
Ipamorelin	Stimulates GH for fat burning	Targeted fat loss, preserving muscle	Targets visceral belly fat without hunger spikes	Requires consistent use
CJC-1295	Extends GH release (longer half-life)	Sustained GH support, stacking protocols	Works synergistically with Ipamorelin	Less effective solo
CJC-1295 + Ipamorelin	GH release combo: sharp + sustained	Fat loss + muscle retention	Synergistic "GH pulse" for sculpting	Requires strategic timing
GHRP-2	GH stimulator without increasing hunger	Leaning without appetite spike	Great during cutting or maintenance	May be milder than GHRP-6
GHRP-6	GH stimulator + appetite booster	Bulking phase or weight gain goals	Increases hunger—great for hard gainers	Not ideal for cutting

Strategic Protocols: Weight Loss Peptide Programs

Beginner Protocols

Starting with peptides can feel like stepping into a new realm of possibilities for weight management. For beginners, simplicity is key. Single-peptide starter regimens allow you to introduce your body gradually to these powerful compounds. A low-dose approach is recommended to observe how your body responds without overwhelming it.

Begin with peptides like Semaglutide, which have proven efficacy in managing appetite and promoting weight loss. Monitor key parameters such as changes in appetite, energy levels, and any side effects. This helps in adjusting the regimen to your specific needs while ensuring safe practices.

Intermediate Strategies

As you gain experience, intermediate strategies open up more advanced opportunities. Synergistic peptide pairings can enhance results by targeting different pathways simultaneously. Combining peptides like Ipamorelin and CJC-1295 can offer enhanced growth hormone release, promoting fat loss and muscle retention.

Cycling methodologies become relevant here, allowing periods of use followed by breaks to maintain efficacy and reduce desensitization. Progress assessment metrics, such as body composition analyses and performance metrics, guide adjustments and ensure alignment with your goals.

Advanced Protocols

Breaking through plateaus requires sophisticated approaches known as advanced protocols. Strategic peptide stacking involves combining multiple peptides to target stubborn fat areas and enhance overall metabolic rate. Pulsed dosing can optimize the body's response by delivering peptides at strategic intervals.

Integrating these with advanced nutritional strategies, such as carb cycling or intermittent fasting, can further amplify results. These methods require meticulous planning and might need professional guidance to ensure safety and effectiveness.

Duration and Cycling

Peptide use isn't a one-size-fits-all solution; understanding duration and cycling recommendations is crucial for sustainable weight management. Short-term protocols might suit those seeking rapid results, while long-term approaches focus on gradual, sustainable changes. Off-cycle strategies are essential to give your body time to recalibrate, reducing the risk of side effects or tolerance build-up. During maintenance phases, consider reduced dosages to preserve gains without the intensity of active weight loss protocols.

Peptides offer a dynamic tool for weight management when used thoughtfully. From beginners to advanced users, tailoring strategies ensures that each step is purposeful and aligned with individual goals.

Lifestyle Integration: Maximizing Peptide Weight Loss

Nutritional Optimization

When you're integrating peptides into your weight loss regimen, the right nutrition can amplify their effects. Protein becomes an ally, not just for muscle maintenance but also because it can enhance peptide efficacy. Aim for a diet rich in lean proteins—think chicken, fish, or plant-based options like lentils and quinoa. These proteins support muscle synthesis and help regulate hunger hormones, ensuring your peptides work more efficiently.

Meanwhile, strategic carbohydrate timing can further tip the scales in your favor. Consuming carbs around your workouts provides the energy needed for peak performance, while keeping intake low during sedentary periods encourages fat metabolism. Micronutrients shouldn't be overlooked either. Vitamins and minerals, from magnesium to B vitamins, play a role in metabolic processes that peptides influence, so eating a varied diet rich in vegetables and fruits is key.

Exercise Synergy

Exercise acts as a catalyst in your weight loss efforts with peptides. Resistance training boosts muscle mass, which directly influences metabolic rate, making it a powerful partner to peptide use. Focus on compound movements like squats and deadlifts; these exercises engage multiple muscle groups, optimizing calorie burn and growth hormone release.

Cardio isn't to be neglected either. Short, intense bursts of activity, such as high-intensity interval training (HIIT), elevate your heart rate and enhance fat oxidation, working harmoniously with peptides' fat-mobilizing properties. Remember, recovery is crucial. Incorporate rest days and consider activities like yoga or stretching to facilitate muscle repair and stress reduction.

Timing Strategies

Timing is everything, particularly when it comes to administering peptides. For pre-workout benefits, consider taking peptides that boost energy and metabolism about 30 minutes before you exercise. Post-workout administration can aid recovery and muscle repair, ensuring you bounce back faster for your next session.

Aligning peptide intake with meals can also optimize absorption and reduce potential side effects. For those targeting better sleep and recovery overnight, incorporating peptides that support relaxation before bedtime can improve sleep quality, enhancing overall results.

Lifestyle Factors

Lifestyle habits significantly impact peptide effectiveness. Managing stress levels is critical; chronic stress disrupts hormonal balance and can counteract peptide benefits. Techniques such as meditation or deep-breathing exercises can help maintain equilibrium.

Prioritizing sleep is equally vital since restorative sleep enhances peptide function and overall recovery. Lastly, be mindful of environmental factors—limiting exposure to toxins or pollutants supports your body's natural detoxification processes, ensuring peptides work efficiently.

Transformation Stories: Weight Loss Success Through Peptides

Clinical Success Stories

In medical practices across the globe, clinicians witness firsthand the transformative potential of peptides. Take the case of severe obesity management, where a patient who struggled for years found new hope through clinically supervised peptide therapy. This approach not only facilitated significant weight loss but also improved their overall metabolic health.

Metabolic syndrome, characterized by a cluster of conditions like high blood pressure and excess body fat around the waist, saw improvement in another patient. Through targeted peptide use, this individual managed to stabilize their blood glucose levels and reduce waist circumference effectively. Even more inspiring are the long-term maintenance success stories where individuals maintain their weight loss with continued peptide support, showing that this isn't just a temporary fix but a sustainable lifestyle change.

Fitness Community Transformations

In the fitness community, enthusiasts embrace peptides as a key element in their transformation arsenal. From body composition improvements, where individuals sculpt their physiques with precision, to contest preparation where athletes achieve peak condition without sacrificing muscle mass, peptides play a pivotal role. Enhanced athletic performance, too, is a common outcome as peptides help improve recovery times and boost energy levels, allowing these athletes to push boundaries they once thought impossible.

Metabolic Health Improvements

Peptides also shine when it comes to metabolic health improvement. Insulin resistance reversal is one such story, where a user managed to enhance insulin sensitivity, reducing their dependence on medication. Cardiovascular health sees similar benefits; peptides help lower cholesterol levels and improve arterial health, contributing to better heart function. Inflammatory markers, often elevated in chronic conditions, are reduced significantly with peptide use, leading to decreased joint pain and improved mobility.

Key Success Factors

Drawing lessons from these successful users reveals common themes. Consistency in peptide use, tailored protocols to fit personal goals, and integration with diet and exercise emerge as success factors. Challenges such as initial side effects are often managed through dose adjustments and professional guidance. Users learn that patience is vital; results unfold over realistic timelines, teaching them that persistence pays off.

As we wrap up this chapter, it's clear that peptides offer a powerful tool for weight management and overall health improvement. These stories show that with the right approach, peptides can lead to profound transformations. Next, we'll explore how peptides contribute to unlocking strength and enhancing recovery, delving into the world of muscle optimization.

Chapter Five

Brain Boosters

Peptides for Cognitive Enhancement

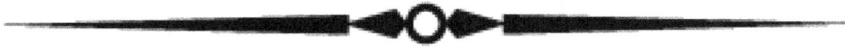

———————◆○◆———————

Mind-Body Connection: How Peptides Enhance Brain Function

O ne quiet evening, I found myself at a personal crossroads. My mind felt foggy—drifting of peptides to enhance cognitive performance and emotional balance.

Though microscopic, peptides exert profound effects on the brain by regulating neurotransmitters—the brain's chemical messengers responsible for focus, mood, and mental agility.

Boosting Brainpower: Peptides and Neurotransmitters

Peptides influence synaptic plasticity, the brain's ability to adapt and reorganize itself. This adaptability is crucial for:

- Learning new skills

- Strengthening memory

- Staying mentally sharp as we age

By enhancing communication between neurons—like upgrading the brain's internal Wi-Fi—certain peptides support faster thinking and deeper recall.

Cerebrolysin & Dihexa: Cognitive Allies

Among the most promising brain-boosting peptides are:

Cerebrolysin – Offers neuroprotection, guards against oxidative stress, and supports cell survival, making it a potential ally in preventing cognitive decline.

Dihexa – Known for its synaptogenic properties, Dihexa promotes the growth of new synapses and enhances the formation of neural pathways. This has exciting implications for memory, focus, and mental clarity. Dihexa has demonstrated strong neuroprotective properties in preclinical trials, improving synaptic connectivity and cognitive function [22].

Mood, Anxiety, and Emotional Regulation

Peptides also support mental well-being by modulating key neurotransmitters:

- Boosting serotonin and dopamine levels

- Reducing symptoms of anxiety and depression

- Stabilizing emotional responses during stress or cognitive overload

This makes them valuable tools not just for performance, but for emotional resilience and everyday peace of mind.

What the Science Says

Clinical studies support the use of peptides in cognitive health. Research highlights improvements in:

- Memory recall

- Focus and attention

- Potential treatment of neurodegenerative diseases through slowed progression and neuroprotection [21]

Peptides not only impact cognition but also influence mood and mental well-being. They can alleviate symptoms of anxiety and depression by modulating neurotransmitter systems involved in these conditions. For instance, peptides can enhance serotonin and dopamine levels, leading to improved mood and reduced anxiety symptoms. This makes them appealing options for individuals dealing with mood disorders.

Scientific studies lend credibility to these claims. Clinical trials have shown that peptides can enhance cognitive performance, improving attention and memory recall [23]. Research also highlights their potential in addressing neurodegenerative diseases by slowing progression and supporting neurological health [24]. These findings underscore the transformative role peptides can play in brain health.

Interactive Element: Reflection Exercise

Consider tracking your mental well-being and cognitive performance over a month. Note any changes in focus or mood when using peptides. This exercise offers valuable insights into how these molecules work for you personally.

By understanding the neurobiological pathways peptides influence, you can appreciate their potential to enhance brain function and support mental health.

Mental Sharpeners: Focus and Memory Peptides

Imagine a world where your mind is as sharp as a tack, slicing through daily challenges with ease. Peptides like Noopept and Semax are your allies in this realm of cognitive enhancement.

Noopept: The Memory Consolidator

Noopept is renowned for memory consolidation, acting like a diligent librarian, organizing information in your brain for easy retrieval. These peptides work by increasing acetylcholine release, a neurotransmitter crucial for learning and memory. They also modulate brain-derived neurotrophic factor (BDNF), a protein that supports neuron growth and connectivity.

Semax: The Concentration Enhancer

Semax, on the other hand, is your go-to for improved concentration, keeping distractions at bay and allowing you to zero in on tasks at hand.

How They Work at the Molecular Level

In the molecular theatre, these peptides shine by enhancing cognitive processes. They boost acetylcholine, which plays a pivotal role in memory and attention. By promoting BDNF, they foster an environment where neurons thrive, akin to nurturing a garden for optimal growth. This biochemical synergy translates into tangible benefits in real-world scenarios.

Real-World Applications

Students in academic settings find their focus sharpened during late-night study sessions. Professionals in high-pressure environments report a newfound clarity, navigating complex problems with precision.

Safety Considerations

Yet, like any tool, these peptides come with guidelines to ensure safe use. Dosage recommendations are crucial to avoid overstimulation. Begin with lower doses and gradually adjust, always monitoring how your body responds. Overuse can lead to headaches or irritability, so it's wise to stay vigilant for any adverse reactions and consult a healthcare provider if needed. Remember that balance is key.

Real-world applications abound for these cognitive enhancers. In academic settings, students find their focus sharpened during those grueling study marathons. Meanwhile, professionals in high-pressure work environments report newfound clarity and the ability to navigate complex problems with precision. However, like any tool, these peptides require careful use. Dosage recommendations are crucial to avoid overstimulation, as too much can lead to headaches or irritability. Starting with lower doses and gradually adjusting is wise, ensuring you monitor how your body responds. If adverse reactions occur, consulting a healthcare provider is recommended.

Calm Creator: Selank- The Anti-Anxiety Peptide

Origins and Development

Selank is a peptide that emerged from the quest to create a new class of anxiolytic (anti-anxiety) compounds, offering a beacon of hope for those battling anxiety. Derived from tuftsin, an immune molecule, Selank was initially developed to combat anxiety, offering an innovative approach to mental health. Tuftsin plays a vital role in modulating immune responses [25], and by building on its structure, researchers crafted Selank to target anxiety more effectively. Gene expression studies suggest that Selank influences neurotransmitter balance and stress response regulation [26]. This peptide has carved a niche for itself by offering a unique mechanism to calm the mind without the sedative effects common in traditional anxiety treatments.

Mechanism of Action

At a molecular level, Selank operates by modulating serotonin and dopamine pathways. These neurotransmitters are crucial for regulating mood and emotional responses. By enhancing their balance, Selank helps foster an internal environment where anxiety struggles to take root. Moreover, it influences GABAergic pathways, which are pivotal in calming neural activity. This modulation promotes a sense of relaxation and well-being, akin to the effects of benzodiazepines but without their side effects.

Clinical Applications

Clinically, Selank has shown promise in treating generalized anxiety disorder (GAD). It provides stress resilience, allowing individuals to navigate daily pressures with greater ease. Those who use Selank often report not just reduced anxiety but also improved mood stability. Unlike some medications that can leave users feeling detached or dulled, Selank maintains mental clarity, making it an attractive option for those seeking effective anxiety relief.

Real-World Impact

Real-world experiences illuminate its impact. Patients with chronic anxiety have shared testimonials of newfound calmness and focus. Quantitative measures show significant reductions in anxiety scores over time, underscoring Selank's potential as a therapeutic tool. For instance, one user noted that their anxiety attacks decreased in frequency and intensity within weeks of starting Selank. Another highlighted enhanced emotional resilience during stressful periods. These stories reinforce the peptide's role as a transformative agent in mental health care, providing real relief where other treatments may fall short.

But remember, while Selank offers substantial benefits, it's essential to approach its use thoughtfully, under professional guidance, ensuring optimal results and safety.

Focus Enhancer: Semax- The Cognitive Booster

Background and Origins

Semax, a peptide developed from adrenocorticotropic hormone (ACTH) fragments, has carved a niche for itself in the realm of cognitive enhancement. Originally from Russia, it has gained popularity as a nootropic and neuroprotective agent, offering a unique approach to boosting mental faculties. While ACTH is primarily known for regulating stress responses, the derivatives used in Semax focus on enhancing cognitive function without the typical stress-related side effects.

How Semax Works

The mechanism by which Semax operates is fascinating. It boosts brain-derived neurotrophic factor (BDNF), a key protein that supports the survival and growth of neurons. BDNF plays a critical role in memory and learning processes, essentially acting as a fertilizer for the brain's neural networks. Moreover, Semax modulates dopaminergic and serotonergic systems, which are vital for maintaining mood stability and enhancing mental clarity. By regulating these neurotransmitters, Semax helps improve focus and attention span, making it a valuable tool for anyone looking to sharpen their cognitive edge.

Applications and Benefits

In terms of applications and benefits, Semax has shown promise in treating cognitive disorders. It supports mental clarity and focus, providing users with an enhanced ability to process information and react swiftly. Whether you're tackling complex tasks at work or diving into new learning opportunities, Semax can offer that extra boost of mental sharpness. Its neuroprotective properties also make it beneficial for long-term brain health, potentially slowing cognitive decline associated with aging.

Scientific Evidence

Comparative studies have placed Semax alongside traditional nootropics, revealing its competitive edge. In trials focusing on memory and attention span enhancement, Semax consistently demonstrated efficacy comparable to or exceeding other cognitive enhancers. Participants reported improved memory recall and sustained attention, underscoring its potential as a leading nootropic. These results highlight Semax's role as a potent cognitive booster, offering tangible benefits that can enhance everyday mental performance.

The data from these studies not only solidifies Semax's standing among cognitive enhancers but also provides a compelling reason for its inclusion in any mental optimization regimen. Its ability to enhance brain function while protecting against cognitive decline makes it an appealing choice for those seeking to maintain or elevate their cognitive abilities.

Wellness clinics now widely offer nootropic peptides like Selank and Semax to support focus and emotional stability [27].

Synergy Stacks: Combining Peptides with Nootropics

The Power of Combination

Imagine the potential of combining peptides with nootropics—two powerhouses working in tandem to elevate your cognitive game. This concept of stacking is gaining traction among biohackers and health enthusiasts alike.

Effective Combinations

Picture pairing Aniracetam with Semax. Aniracetam, a well-known nootropic, boosts memory and learning, while Semax enhances focus and mood. Together, they create a symphony of mental clarity, allowing you to tackle complex tasks with ease. Then consider Ashwagandha, an adaptogenic herb celebrated for its stress-reducing properties. When combined with peptides, it offers a calming effect, making your mental environment more resilient against stressors.

Benefits of Integration

The benefits of this integrated approach are numerous. Enhanced memory retention is one standout advantage. By combining these compounds, you tap into multiple pathways that reinforce each other, leading to more robust memory formation and retrieval. Improved stress resilience is another key benefit. Peptides can modulate neurotransmitters to stabilize mood, while nootropics like Ashwagandha offer additional support by reducing cortisol levels, the stress hormone that can wreak havoc on mental health.

Safety Guidelines

Safety in stacking is paramount. Start by understanding recommended dosages for each component. For instance, begin with low doses of Aniracetam and Semax, observing how your body responds before gradually increasing. Timing is also crucial to avoid tolerance buildup. Consider alternating days or cycles to keep your system responsive. Always prioritize balance and avoid overloading your receptors.

Personalized Protocols

Personalized protocols make all the difference. Each individual's cognitive goals and body chemistry are unique, so tailoring your stack is vital. If you're targeting focus and memory, your combination might differ from someone aiming to reduce anxiety. Consulting with healthcare professionals ensures that your approach is both safe and effective, providing insights tailored to your specific needs.

In this realm of cognitive enhancement, the synergy between peptides and nootropics offers a promising path. By thoughtfully combining these compounds, you can unlock new levels of mental acuity and emotional stability, paving the way for a sharper, more resilient mind.

Mind Masters: Cognitive Enhancement Success Stories

The Software Engineer's Transformation

Imagine the simplicity of a daily routine, now enhanced by the power of peptides. Consider a professional, a software engineer, who struggled with mental fatigue during demanding projects. She turned to Semax, seeking clarity amidst chaos. Within weeks, her focus sharpened, and her productivity soared. The brain fog that once clouded her thoughts lifted, replaced by a crisp mental acuity that allowed her to excel. Her story isn't just about immediate transformation—it highlights the significance of consistency. Regular peptide use became her secret weapon, maintaining cognitive health over time. This isn't a quick fix; it's a long-term strategy.

The University Student's Academic Success

Then there's the tale of a university student facing the daunting challenge of finals. Overwhelmed by the sheer volume of material, he found solace in peptides like Noopept. With diligent use, his study sessions became more effective. Grades improved, not because he studied harder, but because he studied smarter. This student's success underscores the integral role of lifestyle in maximizing peptide benefits. Balanced nutrition and adequate sleep complemented his regimen, amplifying outcomes beyond the peptides alone.

Visual Evidence of Progress

Visual aids can bridge understanding. Imagine graphs depicting cognitive test scores before and after peptide use, illustrating tangible improvements. Infographics can further demystify peptide mechanisms—how they enhance neurotransmission and support brain health—a picture often speaks louder than words.

Key Takeaways

These stories are more than just anecdotes; they're blueprints for potential change. They inspire by showing real possibilities and offer practical insights. Consistency is key for long-term success, and lifestyle factors—like diet and sleep—play a crucial role in maximizing peptide efficacy. By understanding these lessons, you can explore your own cognitive enhancement journey.

As we conclude this chapter on cognitive enhancement with peptides, remember that these stories are not just about boosting brainpower but about enriching overall quality of life. Peptides offer a unique avenue to unlock mental potential, providing hope and tangible results for those seeking well-being—how peptides can influence physical performance and recovery, paving the way for a balanced and vibrant life.

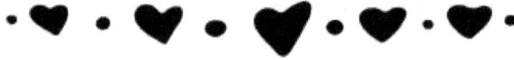

• ♥ • ♥ • ♥ • ♥ • ♥ •

Hi there!

You've reached the midpoint of your peptide optimization journey—well done!

If this book has clarified confusing concepts, helped you feel more confident about peptide safety, or given you actionable protocols to try, I'd love to hear about it.

Your feedback doesn't just mean the world to me—it helps:

- Future readers discover science-based peptide guidance when they need it most

- Me understand which protocols and safety tips resonate most with readers

- Shape improvements for future editions and additional resources

What you share could inspire someone else to start their own journey toward safe, effective health optimization.

Take a quick moment to share your thoughts: Leave Your Review Here

Even just a few sentences about your experience so far would be incredibly valuable!

Thank you for prioritizing evidence-based health optimization!

Warmly,

Sawsan Charif

"Optimal results come not from the peptides you choose, but from how well you understand their purpose, function, and fit for your body."

• ♥ • ♥ • ♥ • ♥ • ♥ •

Chapter Six

Time Reversers

Peptides for Anti-Aging and Longevity

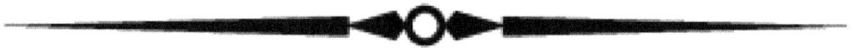

Youth Revolution: Peptides at the Anti-Aging Frontier

I magine standing at the edge of a new era in health—where aging is no longer an unavoidable decline, but a process you can actively manage. That's the promise of peptides: small but mighty molecules that stimulate repair, regeneration, and renewal at the cellular level.

Rewiring the Clock with Telomeres

Peptides play a pivotal role in maintaining telomere length—those protective caps at the ends of chromosomes that prevent genetic damage. As telomeres shorten over time, aging accelerates. But peptides like Epithalon have been shown to activate telomerase, the enzyme that helps rebuild these caps, potentially delaying aging at its source [28].

Among these powerful molecules, Epithalon stands out for its ability to rejuvenate cells by encouraging telomerase activity.

Thymosin Alpha-1: Immunity & Longevity

Another age-defying ally is Thymosin Alpha-1, a peptide that:

- Strengthens immune defenses

- Fights off age-related illness

- Enhances resilience to stress and infection

A robust immune system is a key component of graceful aging, and Thymosin Alpha-1 helps preserve that vitality [29].

DNA Repair and Oxidative Stress Reduction

Peptides also:

- Stimulate DNA repair mechanisms

- Reduce oxidative stress, which damages cells and accelerates the aging process

- Help detoxify at the mitochondrial level for long-term cellular health

By supporting these vital processes, peptides become central to a longevity strategy, not just a short-term supplement.

Backed by Research

Studies on Epithalon show:

- Increased lifespan in animal models

- Improvements in biological markers of aging

- Potential for extending both lifespan and healthspan [30]

Peptides like Epithalon and Thymosin Alpha-1 aren't hype—they're rooted in real, emerging science that targets the foundations of aging itself.

Reflection Prompt

How can you incorporate anti-aging peptides into your wellness routine?

Take a moment to reflect on your current habits. What changes could you make now to support long-term vitality?

Peptides represent a promising frontier in the quest for extended youthfulness. By understanding their mechanisms and incorporating them wisely into our lives, we can embrace aging as an opportunity for growth rather than decline.

Skin Rejuvenator: GHK-Cu - The Copper Peptide

Discovery and Background

GHK-Cu stands as a remarkable agent in skin rejuvenation, a testament to the wonders of modern biochemistry. This copper peptide was discovered in the 1970s, and its unique biochemical structure has captivated the scientific community ever since. Naturally occurring in human plasma, GHK-Cu plays a pivotal role in skin health. Its discovery marked a significant milestone, highlighting its potential to not only repair but rejuvenate the skin, offering a glimpse into the future of dermatological care.

Mechanisms of Action

The mechanisms of GHK-Cu are as fascinating as they are effective. Acting as a robust antioxidant, it reduces oxidative stress, a major culprit in skin aging. By neutralizing free radicals, it shields the skin from environmental damage. Moreover, GHK-Cu enhances wound healing and tissue remodeling by promoting collagen production, pivotal for maintaining skin integrity. It also stimulates glycosaminoglycan synthesis, which aids in retaining moisture and improving skin hydration. These actions collectively contribute to skin rejuvenation, offering both aesthetic and functional benefits. GHK-Cu not only improves skin quality but also modulates numerous cellular pathways related to regeneration and inflammation [31].

Clinical Benefits

Clinically, GHK-Cu has demonstrated significant anti-aging benefits. Users often notice a reduction in fine lines and wrinkles, as well as enhanced skin elasticity and tone. These improvements aren't just superficial; they reflect the peptide's ability to bolster skin health from within. Its efficacy in clinical settings underscores its role as a powerful tool in combating the visible signs of aging.

Application Guidelines

When incorporating GHK-Cu into your skincare regimen, certain considerations enhance its effectiveness. Products with a concentration of 0.1% to 2% are typically recommended for noticeable results. Combining GHK-Cu with other active ingredients like retinol or vitamin C can create a synergistic effect, amplifying its benefits [32]. To maximize impact, ensure consistent application and monitor your skin's response, adjusting usage as needed for optimal outcomes.

Life Extenders: Longevity Peptides Explained

Understanding Longevity vs. Anti-Aging

Longevity, in the context of peptides, shifts the focus from merely adding years to truly enriching those years with health and vitality. It's about enhancing your healthspan—the period of life where you remain active and free from disease. This differs from general anti-aging, which often targets cosmetic concerns.

Longevity emphasizes vitality, especially crucial for aging populations where maintaining an active lifestyle is paramount.

Key Longevity Peptides

Peptides like MOTS-c and Humanin stand out as champions in this arena. MOTS-c optimizes metabolic function, ensuring your body uses energy efficiently, while Humanin protects mitochondria, the powerhouses of your cells, safeguarding them against age-related decline [33].

Cellular Health Benefits

These peptides bolster cellular health in profound ways. They enhance mitochondrial efficiency, making sure every cell runs like a well-oiled machine. This efficiency prevents the tiresome drag of fatigue that often accompanies aging. Additionally, they promote autophagy—your body's natural cleanup process. By clearing out cellular debris, they ensure that cells function optimally, reducing the risk of age-related diseases. This cellular housekeeping is critical for longevity, keeping your body's internal environment pristine.

Implementation Strategy

Incorporating these peptides into your routine requires some thought. Dosages need to be sustainable—too high and you risk imbalances, too low and benefits dwindle. Start with moderate amounts, adjusting based on how your body responds over time. Timing matters too; consider taking MOTS-c in the morning to kickstart your metabolism or Humanin in the evening for recovery. Consistent use is key to reaping long-term benefits.

While these peptides offer promising avenues for extending vitality, remember they should complement a healthy lifestyle. Regular exercise, balanced nutrition, and stress management all play supportive roles. Together with peptides, these practices create a synergy that amplifies your health efforts, paving the way for not just longer life, but a more vibrant one.

Telomere Protector: Epitalon - The Longevity Peptide

Background and Significance

Epitalon, a peptide developed by Russian researchers, stands as a beacon in longevity science. Its significance lies in its ability to regulate the pineal gland, a small but mighty part of your brain involved in sleep and aging processes. By activating telomerase, Epitalon helps maintain telomere length, those protective caps on your DNA strands that naturally shorten with age. This function is crucial because short telomeres are linked to aging and age-related diseases. Additionally, Epitalon influences circadian rhythms, which are your body's internal clock, helping stabilize sleep patterns and overall vitality.

Impact on Lifespan and Vitality

The impact of Epitalon on lifespan and vitality is profound. By promoting telomerase activation, it contributes to telomere elongation, slowing down the cellular aging process. This peptide also plays a role in regulating circadian rhythms, ensuring that your body functions optimally throughout the day. These combined actions not only support longevity but also enhance your quality of life as you age.

Scientific Evidence

Scientific exploration has illuminated Epitalon's potential effects on longevity. Animal studies reveal significant lifespan increases, suggesting its potential as a life-extending treatment. Human trials indicate it may mitigate age-related diseases, offering hope for those seeking to maintain health as they grow older. These studies provide a foundation of evidence supporting Epitalon's role in promoting a longer, healthier life. Studies show Epitalon can activate telomerase and lengthen telomeres, offering potential anti-aging benefits [34].

Practical Application

Incorporating Epitalon into your longevity strategy involves understanding its practical application. Suggested dosing regimens typically involve cycles lasting ten days, repeated several times a year. Timing is essential; many find evening doses beneficial due to Epitalon's influence on circadian rhythms. Cycling ensures that your body remains responsive, maximizing benefits without overwhelming your system. Engaging in regular health monitoring while using Epitalon is wise, offering insights into its effects and ensuring safe use. This approach allows you to harness the power of Epitalon effectively, positioning it as a valuable ally in your quest for extended vitality and youthful living.

Holistic Approach: Integrating Peptides with Longevity Practices

The Symphony of Synergy

The synergy of peptides with other longevity practices is like a finely tuned orchestra, each element playing its part to create a harmonious balance that enhances healthspan and vitality. Consider the integration of peptides with caloric restriction and intermittent fasting. These dietary strategies have shown promise in promoting cellular repair and boosting metabolic efficiency. When combined with peptides, these effects can be amplified, potentially offering greater resilience against age-related decline.

Complementary Practices

Adaptogens and antioxidants also complement peptides, providing a defense against oxidative stress and supporting homeostasis. This combination helps maintain energy levels and fosters a robust internal environment.

Incorporating peptides into a broader longevity strategy can feel like assembling an intricate puzzle where each piece enhances the picture of health. Picture combining peptides with practices like caloric restriction or intermittent fasting. These dietary approaches are not just about cutting calories but about stimulating pathways that can enhance cellular repair and metabolism. When you pair them with peptides, you might amplify these benefits, pushing the boundaries of what each can achieve alone. Adaptogens, known for their stress-reducing properties, also pair well with peptides. Together, they create a robust defense against the wear and tear of daily life by balancing cortisol levels and supporting cellular resilience.

Lifestyle Factors

Lifestyle factors play a critical role in maximizing the benefits of longevity peptides. Regular physical activity is not just about maintaining muscle tone; it promotes cardiovascular health and enhances circulation, ensuring that peptides reach their target sites efficiently. Stress management techniques, such as meditation or yoga, further bolster peptide efficacy by stabilizing hormonal balances and reducing inflammation. These practices create a fertile ground for peptides to exert their rejuvenating effects, enabling a more comprehensive approach to aging well.

Consistent physical activity does more than build muscle; it improves circulation, ensuring peptides reach their target efficiently. Stress management techniques, like meditation, contribute to hormonal balance, enhancing peptide efficacy. Picture these practices as fertile soil, ready to nurture the seeds of peptide action. The synergy between these elements can create a thriving environment for longevity.

Success Stories

Consider the personal stories of individuals who've embraced this holistic approach. Take Jane, for example, who integrated peptides into her routine alongside regular exercise and mindful eating. She reports feeling more energetic and vibrant than ever, attributing her newfound vitality to the seamless blend of modern science and traditional wisdom. Stories from longevity-focused clinics echo these experiences, with clients enjoying enhanced energy levels and improved overall well-being.

Take John, who combined peptides with a regular exercise regimen and mindful eating. He reports feeling more energetic and youthful than ever. At longevity-focused clinics, clients often share their enhanced vitality and well-being, attributing their success to a balanced blend of modern science and traditional wisdom.

Personalized Approach

Viewing peptides as part of a broader health strategy is crucial. Balancing modern medicine with traditional wellness practices encourages personalized longevity plans tailored to individual needs. This approach not only maximizes benefits but also respects the complexity of human health, fostering a sustainable path toward aging with vitality and grace.

Viewing peptides as just one part of a broader health strategy is crucial. Balancing contemporary medicine with age-old wellness practices fosters personalized longevity plans tailored to individual needs. This approach doesn't just maximize benefits; it respects the complexity of human health, offering a sustainable path toward aging with vitality.

Risk-Benefit Balance: Safety in Anti-Aging Peptide Use

Understanding the Risks

As you explore anti-aging peptides, it's crucial to weigh the potential risks against the benefits. These peptides hold promise, but they can also upset hormonal balances, leading to unforeseen complications. There's a chance of unintended cellular proliferation, which could potentially increase the risk of cancer. It's important to be aware of these risks as you consider integrating peptides into your routine. Regular health monitoring and assessments are essential for catching any adverse effects early. Start with lower dosages to gauge how your body reacts before gradually increasing, ensuring you minimize any unwanted side effects.

Ethical Considerations

Ethical considerations also play a significant role in the pursuit of longevity through peptides. Extending lifespans raises societal questions: What happens when lifespans extend far beyond what's considered normal? How do we ensure that everyone has access to these advancements? Furthermore, ethical sourcing and production of peptides are critical. Sustainable practices in peptide manufacturing must be emphasized to prevent harm to the environment and ensure fair labor conditions.

The Need for Continued Research

The field of anti-aging peptides is still burgeoning, making continued research imperative. Scientific exploration and innovation drive this field forward, providing new insights and improving peptide efficacy and safety. I encourage you to stay informed about new discoveries and advancements. Engaging in or supporting research studies can contribute to the collective understanding of these potent molecules.

In wrapping up this chapter, it's clear that while anti-aging peptides offer exciting possibilities, they aren't without risks. Balancing benefits with potential downsides requires vigilance and informed decision-making. As we move forward, let's keep an eye on the future of longevity science, mindful of both ethical considerations and the need for continued research. Next, we'll explore how these peptides can intersect with physical performance, offering insights into enhancing not just lifespan but life quality as well.

Chapter Seven

Skin Saviors

Skin Science: How Peptides Transform Your Complexion

Imagine waking up to a complexion that radiates health and vitality. This isn't just wishful thinking—it's possible thanks to peptides. These tiny yet powerful molecules have become heroes in the skincare world, celebrated for their ability to restore, rebuild, and rejuvenate.

Collagen Production & Skin Firmness

Peptides act as messengers within your skin, stimulating natural collagen production—a key player in maintaining firmness and elasticity. Think of them as conductors in a symphony, guiding your skin's regenerative rhythms and keeping it plump and youthful.

Strengthening the Skin Barrier

Peptides also help fortify the skin's protective barrier, shielding against:

- UV rays

- Pollution

- Environmental stressors

A strong barrier means:
- Better moisture retention

- Fewer irritants penetrating the skin

- A smoother, more radiant surface

It's like turning the dial from dull to dewy.

Calming, Healing, and Rejuvenating

Peptides shine when addressing common skin issues like:
- Fine lines and wrinkles

- Redness and inflammation

- Acne and sensitivity

By reducing inflammation and accelerating cellular repair, peptides help:
- Calm flare-ups

- Speed up healing

- Restore clarity and glow to irritated skin

For those with sensitive or acne-prone complexions, peptides offer a gentle yet effective solution.

Beauty Meets Biohacking

Skincare peptides—like GHK-Cu and Palmitoyl Pentapeptide-4—are at the forefront of cosmeceutical innovation. They not only beautify the skin but also biohack its renewal from the inside out.

This fusion of science and self-care makes peptides a core tool in any anti-aging or glow-up routine.

Scientific Evidence

Peptides stand out for their remarkable capacity to address and alleviate common skin issues such as fine lines, wrinkles, acne, redness, and sensitivity. For individuals dealing with sensitive or acne-prone skin, the reduction in inflammation brought about by peptides offers a soothing balm that calms redness and irritated skin, providing much-needed relief. This anti-inflammatory action also aids in clearing blemishes and accelerates the healing process of existing breakouts. With consistent use, you will observe a visible reduction in fine lines and wrinkles as peptides work their magic on refining and smoothing your skin's texture.

Scientific evidence supports these benefits, with numerous studies highlighting peptides' efficacy in skincare. Clinical studies have shown that some peptides can stimulate collagen production by up to 350%, dramatically reducing the appearance of fine lines while improving texture, elasticity, and hydration levels [35]. This research and clinical validation underscores why peptides are more than a fleeting trend—they have established themselves as a cornerstone of modern skincare innovations. Additional research confirms peptides can stimulate skin basement membrane protein expression, further supporting anti-aging effects [36].

Visual Element: Reflection Exercise

Consider keeping a skincare journal dedicated to tracking the changes in your complexion as you engage with peptide-rich products. Document improvements in texture, hydration, resilience, and overall appearance, painting a vivid picture of progress over time. This practice not only empowers you to witness transformation but also allows you to tailor your skincare routine, optimizing results for your skin's unique needs.

Incorporating peptides into your skincare regimen isn't just a step—it's a confident leap towards achieving healthier, more radiant skin. Embrace this journey as an opportunity to nurture and cherish your skin, unleashing its full potential and basking in the beauty of your transformation.

Collagen Commanders: Peptides for Elasticity and Firmness

How Peptides Boost Collagen

Peptides are like skilled operatives, working beneath the surface of your skin to amplify collagen production—crucial for preserving youthful resilience and elasticity. These tiny powerhouses accomplish this by activating fibroblasts, the pivotal cells responsible for synthesizing collagen.

Think of fibroblasts as the architects of your skin; they lay the foundational elements that sustain its structure. By awakening these cells, peptides effectively bolster the natural collagen synthesis process, serving as a sophisticated signal to the body's innate collagen production. It's like providing your skin with a gentle nudge—a reminder to persist in maintaining firmness and resilience. The skin's response to these signals acts like a well-timed tune-up, enhancing its elasticity and vitality.

Key Collagen-Boosting Peptides

Certain peptides have risen to prominence as notable players in collagen enhancement:

Matrixyl – This renowned peptide complex excels at promoting both collagen and elastin production. Together, this potent combination achieves enhanced skin elasticity and firmness, smoothing out fine lines that appear as time progresses.

Palmitoyl Pentapeptide-4 – This peptide fortifies skin structure and supports firmness. Through its ongoing interaction with skin cells, it promotes the production of collagen and other structural proteins essential for maintaining skin integrity.

These peptides are strategic allies in the anti-aging battle, each fulfilling a distinct role in reinforcing your skin's fundamental scaffolding.

Visible Transformation Results

As collagen levels rise and invigorate your skin, the changes become evident—smoother fine lines and a noticeable decrease in wrinkles. Like reinforcing the walls of a castle, your skin structure solidifies with improved support and increased resilience against daily environmental stresses. This rejuvenation creates a lasting youthful appearance that defies time's passage.

Your skin rebounds with newfound energy, regaining its buoyancy and appearing more lifted and full. The results are tangible—not only visible to the eye but perceptible to the touch, evident in the renewed softness that greets your fingertips each morning.

Consistency is Key

Sustaining these outcomes requires dedication and consistent application. Daily use of peptide-enhanced products is crucial, allowing these molecules to integrate seamlessly into your skincare routine. Consistent reinforcement ensures sustained collagen production, promising lasting benefits over time.

For optimal results, consider pairing peptides with other collagen-supportive elements such as hyaluronic acid or vitamin C. The synergy of these ingredients amplifies hydration and shields against free radicals, perfectly complementing peptide action to enhance skin health.

Long-Term Investment

Incorporating peptides into your skincare ritual is like making a substantial investment in your skin's vitality and future well-being. As you consistently nurture your skin with these potent molecules, you're addressing current concerns while laying a robust foundation for skin that retains its resilience, vitality, and youthful glow over the years. Peptides transcend mere skincare ingredients; they emerge as indispensable partners in maintaining elasticity and firmness.

Product Navigator: Finding Effective Peptide Skincare

Understanding the Market

Venturing into the realm of peptide skincare can be both thrilling and overwhelming. The market is brimming with options, each promising to transform your skin. From serums that deliver concentrated active ingredients to creams that provide hydration while infusing peptides deep within the dermis, the variety is vast. Masks offer a luxurious experience, enveloping your skin in a rich blend of peptides and other nourishing compounds. Many products combine peptides with vitamins, antioxidants, and hyaluronic acid, each component working synergistically to enhance efficacy.

Choosing Quality Products

Choosing the right peptide product requires discernment. Focus on reputable brands known for transparency and integrity. Brands that readily disclose ingredient lists and provide evidence of clinical testing demonstrate a commitment to quality. Look for formulations that highlight clinically tested benefits, as these are more likely to deliver on promises.

Key factors to consider:

- Peptides should be prominent ingredients, not buried at the end of the list

- Concentration matters—higher levels often indicate more potent results

- Trustworthy brands often share research or partner with dermatologists to validate claims

Navigating Marketing Claims

Navigating marketing claims can be tricky. The beauty industry is rife with buzzwords designed to catch attention but often lack substance. Words like "revolutionary" or "miracle" warrant skepticism unless backed by solid scientific evidence. Instead, look for products that emphasize scientifically backed ingredients.

Terms like "clinically proven" or "dermatologist tested" carry weight when accompanied by real data. Be wary of products that promise overnight results or seem too good to be true; skincare is a gradual process, and patience is key. Genuine results come from consistent use of well-researched formulations.

Integration Strategies

Integrating peptide products into your routine requires a thoughtful approach. Consider your skin type and existing regimen when introducing new products. Peptide serums can be applied after cleansing and before moisturizing, allowing them to penetrate deeply.

If you're using other active ingredients like retinol or vitamin C, layering correctly ensures maximum benefit without irritation. For those with sensitive skin, starting with a lower concentration can help your skin adjust without adverse reactions. Adjustments might be necessary based on seasonal changes or specific skin concerns, so stay attuned to how your skin responds.

Skin Type Considerations

Each skin type has unique needs and challenges:

Dry skin – Pair peptides with rich moisturizers to enhance hydration and barrier protection

Oily or acne-prone skin – Benefit from lighter formulations that don't clog pores but still deliver anti-aging benefits

Tailor your routine to address these needs while ensuring peptides play a central role in your skincare strategy. Regularly reassess your skin's condition and adjust your approach as needed, ensuring long-term health and vitality.

Finding the right peptide products is about informed choices—where science meets self-care. It's about being savvy with selections and understanding what genuine transformations look like over time. Embracing a tailored approach allows for optimal results, leading to a complexion that truly reflects the care you invest in it.

Skin Transformations: Real Results with Peptides

Individual Success Stories

In the world of skincare, real stories speak volumes about the transformative potential of peptides.

Sarah's Anti-Aging Journey – Sarah battled with early signs of aging, noticing crow's feet and a dullness that seemed to cast a shadow over her natural glow. By integrating a peptide-rich serum into her routine, she witnessed a rejuvenation that felt like turning back time. Her skin not only looked firmer but also radiated youthful vitality.

Mark's Acne Transformation – Mark faced persistent acne and accompanying redness. With consistent use of peptides known for calming inflammation, Mark found his complexion clearing and his confidence soaring.

These stories underscore the promise peptides hold—not just as skincare products, but as catalysts for personal transformation.

Versatility Across Skin Types

Peptides cater to a variety of skin types, illustrating their versatility and broad appeal:

Sensitive Skin – Individuals with sensitive skin often tread cautiously in the skincare aisle, wary of products that might irritate. Yet, peptides offer a soothing solution, enhancing skin resilience without triggering adverse reactions. Emily, whose sensitive skin once reacted to almost every product, found peace in peptide-based formulations that fortified her dermal barrier without causing flare-ups.

Mature Skin – Those with mature skin, like George, appreciate peptides for their role in smoothing wrinkles and restoring elasticity. Palmitoyl Pentapeptide-4, a common cosmetic peptide, has been shown to support skin elasticity and reduce fine lines [37].

Acne-Prone Skin – Even acne-prone individuals see benefits; peptides help manage oil production and reduce inflammation, leading to clearer skin over time.

Common Success Factors

Success stories from peptide users reveal common threads:

Patience and Consistency – Users who achieve the best results understand that skincare is a marathon, not a sprint. Regular application allows peptides to work gradually, leading to sustainable improvements.

Personalized Approaches – Tailoring peptide use to specific needs—whether targeting fine lines or reducing redness—ensures optimal outcomes. The ability to adapt routines based on individual responses plays a crucial role in achieving desired results.

Visual Evidence

Visual elements like before-and-after photos or progress charts serve as compelling evidence of these transformations. They capture the subtle yet significant changes in skin texture, tone, and overall appearance. Infographics illustrating individual journeys can enhance understanding and engagement, offering a visual roadmap of what's possible with peptide use. These tools not only inspire but also educate, providing clear examples of what effective peptide skincare can achieve.

As we wrap up this chapter on skin transformations, remember that peptides offer more than just aesthetic benefits—they empower individuals to take control of their skincare and embrace their unique beauty. This exploration of skin health sets the stage for our next chapter, where we delve deeper into how peptides can enhance athletic performance and aid recovery. Together, these insights pave the way for holistic well-being and vitality.

Chapter Eight

Athletic Edge

Peptides in Sports Performance

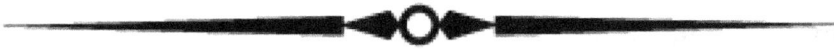

———◆◇◆———

Performance Revolution: The Peptide Advantage in Sports

I magine you're on the field, the track, or in the ring, feeling the exhilaration of pushing your limits. Now imagine having an edge that not only enhances your performance but also accelerates your recovery. This is where peptides come into play, emerging as a significant factor in athletic performance enhancement.

Peptides are short chains of amino acids, the building blocks of proteins, and they have taken the sports world by storm. They offer athletes a means to enhance muscle recovery and repair, improve endurance, and ultimately elevate overall athletic prowess. Unlike traditional methods that often require prolonged recovery periods, peptides offer an innovative solution by reducing downtime and muscle fatigue, enabling athletes to train harder and more frequently.

What Sets Peptides Apart

What sets peptides apart from traditional performance-enhancing methods is their ability to expedite recovery times and reduce muscle fatigue. Traditional supplements may take time to show results, but peptides act swiftly, stimulating muscle protein synthesis and enhancing oxygen delivery to muscles. This means faster recovery from intense workouts and competitions, allowing athletes to maintain peak performance levels consistently.

The science behind this lies in peptides' ability to trigger anabolic pathways that promote muscle growth and repair while simultaneously enhancing endurance through improved blood flow and oxygen transport.

Future Implications

The real-world implications of peptides in sports are vast. As research continues to unfold, the potential for personalized peptide protocols tailored to individual athletes becomes more achievable. Imagine a future where elite athletes integrate these protocols into their training regimens, optimizing every aspect of their performance. This could revolutionize the landscape of sports, allowing athletes to reach new heights safely and effectively.

By understanding the mechanisms at play, athletes can make informed decisions about how best to incorporate peptides into their routines, maximizing their benefits and minimizing risks.

Interactive Element: Personalized Peptide Planning

Consider crafting a personalized peptide plan. Reflect on your specific athletic goals, whether it's improving endurance, enhancing muscle recovery, or increasing overall performance. Jot down which peptides align with these goals and develop a strategy for integrating them into your training regimen. This exercise can serve as a roadmap for incorporating peptides effectively and safely.

As we delve deeper into this chapter, keep in mind that the world of peptides offers untapped potential for athletic performance. With careful consideration and informed choices, you can unlock an athletic edge that propels you toward your goals.

Endurance Enhancers: Peptides for Stamina and Performance

Key Endurance Peptides

When it comes to endurance, some peptides offer extraordinary benefits:

Erythropoietin (EPO) is well-known for increasing red blood cell production, which enhances oxygen delivery to muscles, boosting stamina significantly (Australian Academy of Science, n.d.). Imagine your muscles receiving a constant oxygen supply, allowing them to perform better and recover faster. Erythropoietin (EPO) is well-known for increasing red blood cell production, which enhances oxygen delivery to muscles, boosting stamina significantly [38].

AICAR improves metabolic efficiency by encouraging the body to burn fat instead of carbohydrates as fuel. This shift in metabolism can lead to increased energy levels during prolonged activities like marathons or cycling races.

Performance Benefits

These peptides work wonders for aerobic performance. Enhanced mitochondrial function is a game-changer. Mitochondria, often referred to as the powerhouse of cells, become more efficient at producing energy when boosted by peptides. This results in an increased VO2 max—the maximum amount of oxygen your body can utilize during intense exercise. Simply put, more oxygen equals better performance and endurance. With improved oxygen delivery and utilization, athletes find themselves capable of pushing their limits further than ever before.

Strategic Implementation

Incorporating peptides into endurance training requires strategic planning. Timing is crucial. For instance, administering EPO or AICAR a few hours before a workout can ensure optimal levels during exercise. Combining these peptides with structured endurance programs maximizes benefits. You might consider alternating between high-intensity interval training and long, steady sessions to fully exploit the advantages peptides offer. Keeping a detailed log of your routine helps fine-tune these strategies for even better results.

Potential Challenges

Despite their benefits, using peptides for endurance isn't without challenges. Overuse and dependency are significant risks. Athletes may find themselves tempted to rely solely on peptides for performance boosts, neglecting foundational training principles. To counter this, it's essential to integrate peptides as part of a holistic training plan rather than a standalone solution.

Monitoring for side effects is equally important. Common issues like elevated heart rate or blood pressure can occur if dosage isn't carefully managed. Regular check-ins with health professionals ensure safe use, especially during competitions where stress levels are high.

Athletes looking to enhance their endurance should approach peptide use with a balanced mindset. While the allure of improved performance is undeniable, the foundation should always be sound training and recovery practices. Peptides offer a valuable tool in the athlete's arsenal when used responsibly, enhancing physiological capabilities in ways that were once unimaginable.

Supplement Showdown: Peptides vs. Traditional Options

Performance Comparison

In the world of sports supplements, peptides and traditional options like creatine and branched-chain amino acids (BCAAs) often vie for attention. Peptides have gained popularity due to their targeted action, offering athletes a unique edge. Expert reviews suggest that tailored peptide therapy can optimize recovery and endurance for athletes [39].

Creatine, a staple in bodybuilding, excels in short bursts of muscle growth and power by refueling ATP energy reserves. Peptides, however, provide a more nuanced approach by stimulating muscle repair and protein synthesis at a cellular level. This means not only muscle growth but also enhanced recovery and endurance, broadening their appeal beyond just strength athletes.

Recovery Benefits

When it comes to recovery, **BCAAs** have long been cherished for their role in muscle repair and reducing exercise-induced fatigue. They provide the essential amino acids needed by muscles post-exercise. Peptides, on the other hand, go a step further by influencing hormones and enhancing overall recovery processes. BCAAs offer quick relief, but peptides contribute to long-term gains by promoting cellular health and regeneration. It's a difference between applying a band-aid and actually healing the wound.

While creatine and BCAAs are generally considered safe and legal, peptides offer bioactive advantages that may go beyond muscle repair, including enhanced recovery, metabolism, and cellular signaling [40].

Safety and Legal Considerations

Safety profiles are paramount when choosing supplements. Peptides, being highly specific, often come with fewer side effects compared to traditional supplements. However, their misuse can lead to long-term health impacts, including hormonal imbalances. Contamination risk is also a concern for both peptides and traditional supplements, especially with less reputable brands.

Doping violations loom large in the sports world, with anti-doping agencies keeping a close watch on peptide use due to their performance-enhancing potential. While creatine and BCAAs are generally considered safe and legal, peptides require careful monitoring to avoid crossing ethical lines.

Regulatory Landscape

The regulatory landscape for peptides and traditional supplements is complex. Anti-doping agencies like WADA have stringent guidelines on prohibited substances, with peptides often falling under scrutiny due to their potent effects. Athletes must navigate these regulations carefully to avoid violations. Creatine and BCAAs usually escape such scrutiny, being classified as legal under most sports guidelines. Legal status varies significantly across sports and regions, making it essential for athletes to stay informed about current regulations. While some peptides remain under investigation, many are already popular among athletes and bodybuilders for muscle growth, fat loss, and recovery support [41].

Making the Right Choice

Deciding between peptides and traditional supplements involves a thoughtful process. Athletes should evaluate their personal health goals and sports requirements. Are you looking for quick muscle gain or sustainable performance improvement? Consulting with sports nutritionists and healthcare providers can provide valuable insights tailored to individual needs.

While peptides offer cutting-edge benefits, traditional supplements still hold value for many athletes seeking reliable support without the regulatory complexities. Ultimately, the key lies in informed choices—understanding what each option offers and aligning it with your athletic ambitions.

Champion Profiles: Athletes' Experiences with Peptides

Endurance Success Stories

Imagine the thrill of crossing a finish line, not just completing but conquering, all thanks to the subtle yet potent power of peptides. These little chains of amino acids have quietly revolutionized the way athletes train and perform.

Marathon Runner – One marathon runner who integrated peptides into their regimen reported improved stamina, allowing them to maintain a steady pace throughout grueling races. This wasn't just about finishing faster; it was about feeling powerful, even at the final stretch.

Triathlete – A triathlete noticed a significant reduction in recovery time, enabling more frequent and intense training sessions without the usual fatigue. These athletes' testimonials highlight how peptides can transform endurance training, pushing limits and extending capabilities.

Strength Sport Transformations

For strength athletes, peptides have been game-changers as well:

Powerlifter – One powerlifter who incorporated peptides for muscle repair and growth observed a notable increase in strength and power output over time, breaking personal records and setting new benchmarks, supported by long-term evidence on muscle mass enhancement [42]. The peptides played a crucial role in optimizing their body's anabolic processes, leading to faster muscle recovery and enhanced performance during competitions.

Strength Athlete – Another strength athlete found that peptides reduced their injury rates, keeping them in peak condition year-round. These stories emphasize the tangible benefits that peptides bring to strength sports—enabling athletes to recover quickly, train harder, and achieve greater results.

Key Learning Points

Lessons learned from these athletes provide valuable insights into effective peptide use:

- **Customization is crucial** – The importance of customizing peptide protocols to align with individual goals and needs. What works for one athlete might not work for another.

- **Continuous monitoring** – Ongoing adjustments are essential, allowing athletes to fine-tune their regimens for optimal results.

- **Professional guidance** – Regular consultations with healthcare professionals ensure safety and efficacy, minimizing risks while maximizing benefits.

Performance Visualization

To visualize these achievements, consider performance data visualizations that capture before-and-after metrics. Imagine charts displaying increases in speed or power output, side by side with recovery rates over time. Such visual elements not only engage readers but also offer a concrete understanding of how peptides impact athletic performance.

Through personalized plans and ongoing adjustments, athletes have harnessed peptides to unlock untapped potential. By learning from their successes and challenges, you too can explore how these powerful molecules might enhance your own athletic endeavors.

Ethical Playbook: Navigating Peptides in Competitive Sports

Understanding Regulations

In competitive sports, the line between fair play and gaining an unfair advantage can be thin. This is where doping regulations, such as those set by the World Anti-Doping Agency (WADA), come into play. WADA maintains a prohibited substances list, which includes certain peptides that could unfairly enhance performance [43]. These rules exist to ensure a level playing field, but they also mean athletes need to be acutely aware of what they're putting into their bodies.

Understanding testing methodologies and detection windows is vital. Anti-doping tests can detect banned substances long after use, meaning athletes must be cautious about timing and compliance with these regulations.

Ethical Considerations

Ethical use of peptides in sports is a hot topic. Therapeutic Use Exemptions (TUEs) allow athletes to use certain banned substances if they are medically necessary. However, balancing therapeutic needs with maintaining fairness and competition integrity remains challenging.

The moral question isn't just about following rules but also considering the spirit of sport. Is it fair to use peptides if they give one athlete an edge over another who isn't using them? These considerations form a complex web of ethics that athletes must navigate thoughtfully.

Sport-Specific Regulations

Different sports organizations have varying rules regarding peptide use, making it crucial for athletes to understand the specific regulations of their league. Professional sports may have stricter enforcement compared to amateur leagues. Moreover, sport-specific regulatory differences mean that what is permissible in one discipline might be restricted in another. Athletes must stay updated with their sport's governing body's policies to avoid unintentional violations.

Future Outlook

Looking ahead, the future of peptides in regulated sports is intriguing. Emerging testing technologies promise more accurate detection of peptide use, potentially changing how athletes and regulators view these substances. There's also a conversation about accepting therapeutic applications of peptides in sports, which could lead to broader acceptance under specific guidelines. As the science behind peptides evolves, so too will the rules governing their use, requiring athletes to remain informed and adaptable.

In summary, navigating the ethical landscape of peptide use in sports involves understanding stringent regulations, considering moral implications, and keeping up with changing rules and technologies. Peptides offer significant potential for enhancing athletic performance, but their use must align with the principles of fair play and sportsmanship.

As this chapter concludes, remember that while peptides can enhance physical capabilities, true athletic excellence lies in dedication, discipline, and integrity. In the next chapter, we'll explore how sleep and recovery play crucial roles in achieving optimal performance and longevity.

Chapter Nine

Healing Heroes

Peptides for Recovery and Repair

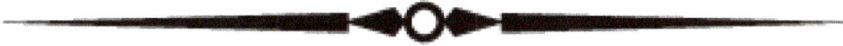

───────◆─○─◆───────

Tissue Mender: TB-500 and Thymosin Beta-4

I magine your body as a dynamic ecosystem, constantly mending and adapting to life's demands. Enter TB-500, a healing peptide with origins deeply rooted in Thymosin Beta-4 (TB4). This peptide, naturally occurring in your body, is a powerhouse for tissue repair and regeneration. Known for its remarkable ability to enhance healing, TB-500 has gained attention for its regenerative properties, especially among athletes and those with chronic injuries. It acts much like a master orchestrator, coordinating the body's repair processes and ensuring everything runs smoothly. Furthermore, this peptide enhances cell migration and differentiation, essential for rebuilding tissues. It encourages cells to move where needed, facilitating rapid repair[33].

Mechanisms of Healing

TB-500's efficacy lies in its mechanisms promoting recovery:

Angiogenesis Stimulation – It stimulates the formation of new blood vessels, which is crucial for delivering oxygen and nutrients to injured tissues. This process accelerates healing by enhancing blood flow to damaged areas.

Anti-Inflammatory Effects – TB-500 reduces inflammation at injury sites, creating an environment conducive to recovery. By curbing inflammation, it alleviates pain and swelling, allowing tissues to heal more efficiently.

Enhanced Cell Migration – This peptide enhances cell migration and differentiation, essential for rebuilding tissues. It encourages cells to move where needed, facilitating rapid repair [44].

Applications and Benefits

In various recovery scenarios, TB-500 shines as an invaluable ally:

- **Sports injury recovery** – A staple in athletic recovery protocols, helping athletes return to peak performance

- **Tendon and muscle injuries** – Whether it's a torn tendon or a strained muscle, TB-500 expedites recovery, reducing downtime significantly

- **Chronic conditions** – Applications extend to treating conditions like arthritis, where its anti-inflammatory properties provide relief and improved joint function

This peptide offers a beacon of hope for those seeking natural solutions to manage long-term pain and stiffness.

Usage Guidelines

When incorporating TB-500 into your recovery regimen, following guidelines for use and safety is crucial:

- **Administration method** – Recommended dosing schedules typically involve subcutaneous injections, which are easy to administer and allow for precise control over dosage

- **Dosage progression** – Dosages usually start small and gradually increase as your body adapts

- **Monitoring** – While generally well-tolerated, some individuals may experience mild redness or irritation at the injection site

- **Professional guidance** – Consult a healthcare professional familiar with peptide therapy to tailor the dosing regimen based on individual needs

Interactive Element: Recovery Reflection Exercise

Consider keeping a recovery journal to track your progress with TB-500. Document your injury details, dosing schedules, and any changes in pain levels or mobility. This practice provides insights into how your body responds to TB-500, helping you fine-tune your regimen for optimal results.

TB-500 stands out as a versatile tool in the recovery toolkit. By understanding its mechanisms and applications, you can leverage its benefits effectively, paving the way for enhanced healing and a return to vitality.

Body Protector: BPC-157 - The Healing Compound

Origins and Discovery

Imagine a compound derived from the very essence of your body's digestive system, playing a pivotal role in recovery. Enter BPC-157, a peptide first discovered as a derivative of gastric juice. This humble origin belies its powerful capabilities. Initially recognized for its role in gut health, BPC-157 has evolved into a therapeutic agent renowned for promoting healing across various bodily systems. It's like having an internal repair crew on standby, ready to jump into action whenever needed.

Healing Mechanisms

BPC-157 works wonders through mechanisms that repair and rejuvenate:

Angiogenesis Enhancement – It stimulates the process of forming new blood vessels, ensuring that injured areas receive ample oxygen and nutrients for recovery. This angiogenic effect is crucial for tissue regeneration, particularly in areas with limited blood supply.

Growth Factor Activation – BPC-157 activates growth factors within the body, accelerating the healing process. By enhancing the production of these factors, it lays the groundwork for efficient repair and recovery. Studies also show that BPC-157 enhances the activity of the growth hormone receptor, further amplifying its healing capabilities [45]. Think of it as providing the building blocks necessary for constructing a robust and resilient body.

Diverse Applications

Its applications are diverse and impressive:

Digestive Health – In the realm of digestive health, BPC-157 shines by repairing gastric and intestinal tissues. It mitigates the damage caused by ulcers and inflammatory conditions, promoting mucosal healing and gastrointestinal balance.

Tendon and Ligament Recovery – For those grappling with tendon or ligament injuries, BPC-157 offers a lifeline. Its ability to facilitate tendon and ligament regeneration has made it a favorite among athletes and active individuals aiming for comprehensive recovery.

Administration Strategies

When it comes to administering BPC-157, strategy is key:

Local Administration – Focuses on injecting the peptide directly into the affected area, targeting specific injuries with precision. This method is especially effective for concentrated healing efforts.

Systemic Administration – Involves a broader approach, allowing the peptide to circulate throughout the body for widespread benefits.

Timing and Cycling – Cycling recommendations suggest periods of use followed by rest to prevent tolerance build-up.

Case Study: A Runner's Return

Consider John, an avid runner sidelined by a stubborn Achilles injury. Incorporating BPC-157 into his recovery plan, he noticed significant improvements in mobility and pain reduction within weeks. This peptide allowed him to gradually return to training without setbacks.

BPC-157's potential is vast, offering hope to those seeking natural healing solutions. By understanding its origins and mechanisms, you can effectively incorporate it into your recovery regimen. Whether it's soothing an inflamed gut or restoring tendon integrity, this peptide stands ready to assist in your journey toward optimal health and vitality.

Immune Guardian: The Power of Thymosin Alpha-1

Background and Discovery

Thymosin Alpha-1 emerges as a beacon of hope in the realm of immune enhancement and recovery. Originally discovered in the 1960s, this peptide has since carved its niche in medical science due to its remarkable ability to modulate the immune response [46]. It's like having an internal coach for your immune system, guiding it to react appropriately to threats. By enhancing the immune system's efficiency, Thymosin Alpha-1 has become a cornerstone for therapies aimed at boosting resilience and accelerating recovery from various health challenges.

Mechanisms of Action

The peptide's potency lies in its mechanisms of action:

T-Cell Enhancement – Particularly its enhancement of T-cell production and activity. T-cells are vital players in the immune response, acting as soldiers that identify and attack invaders. Thymosin Alpha-1 increases their numbers and activity levels, ensuring a robust defense against infections.

Anti-Inflammatory Effects – It reduces pro-inflammatory cytokines—those molecules that contribute to chronic inflammation and tissue damage. This dual action not only fortifies your body's defenses but also creates a more harmonious internal environment conducive to healing.

Clinical Applications

In clinical settings, Thymosin Alpha-1 finds applications across a spectrum of conditions:

- **Infection recovery** – Particularly effective in accelerating recovery from infections and illnesses, helping your body bounce back quicker by strengthening its natural defenses

- **Autoimmune disorders** – Shows promise in managing autoimmune disorders, where it helps regulate the immune system's overactive responses

- **Chronic fatigue** – Those with chronic fatigue syndrome report improved energy levels and overall well-being, underscoring its versatility as an immune booster

Usage Protocols and Safety

Incorporating Thymosin Alpha-1 into your health regimen requires careful consideration:

- **Optimal dosing** – Too little might not offer the desired benefits, while too much could potentially lead to adverse effects

- **Administration** – Typically administered subcutaneously, following prescribed dosing schedules tailored to individual needs

- **Monitoring** – Regular monitoring ensures safety and efficacy, with healthcare providers playing a key role in adjusting dosages based on your body's response

- **Contraindications** – Those with certain medical conditions or who are pregnant should consult a healthcare professional before considering this peptide

Thymosin Alpha-1 stands out as an immune guardian, offering a blend of protection and recovery. By understanding its origins and mechanisms, you can effectively incorporate it into your immune health strategy. Whether you're aiming to bolster your defenses or seeking support for existing conditions, this peptide offers a promising avenue for enhanced resilience and vitality.

Inflammation Fighters: Peptide Solutions for Pain and Swelling

Understanding Inflammation in Recovery

In the realm of injury management, peptides have emerged as potent allies, particularly in managing inflammation. When you're dealing with an injury, it's not just about the initial damage. The subsequent inflammation can be both a hindrance and a help. On one hand, it signals the body to start the repair process. On the other, excessive inflammation can prolong recovery and lead to chronic pain.

This is where specific peptides come into play, offering a targeted approach to reduce inflammation at the cellular level and accelerate tissue regeneration [47].

By modulating inflammatory responses, these peptides ensure a balanced healing environment, minimizing unnecessary swelling while promoting faster recovery.

Key Anti-Inflammatory Peptides

Among the peptides commonly used for injury recovery:

BPC-157 – Stands out particularly for gastrointestinal and tendon injuries. Known for its protective qualities, it aids in repairing damaged tissues by fostering angiogenesis and enhancing cellular communication. Its ability to stabilize and heal makes it indispensable in injury protocols.

KPV – Effective against skin and soft tissue inflammation. It works by targeting inflammatory pathways, making it ideal for reducing redness and swelling in affected areas.

These peptides serve as the body's internal repair crew, addressing specific needs with precision.

Mechanisms of Action

The mechanisms of action in these peptides are fascinating:

- **Pathway inhibition** – They operate by inhibiting key inflammatory pathways that often run rampant post-injury, preventing excessive inflammation that can hinder recovery

- **Anti-inflammatory boost** – They boost the production of anti-inflammatory cytokines—helpful molecules that counteract inflammation and promote healing

- **Balanced response** – This dual action ensures that the body's response remains balanced, allowing tissues to regenerate without the burden of chronic inflammation

It's like having a well-oiled machine where each component works in harmony, ensuring optimal performance.

Integration with Rehabilitation

Integrating peptides into rehabilitation protocols requires a thoughtful approach:

Synergy with Physical Therapy – When combined with physical therapy, peptides can significantly enhance recovery outcomes. Physical therapy mobilizes tissues, and when paired with peptides that reduce inflammation and promote healing, it creates a synergistic effect that accelerates recovery.

Progress Monitoring – Monitoring progress is crucial; adjust peptide dosages based on how your body responds to treatment. This ensures that the healing process is optimized without over-reliance on any single method.

Body Feedback – Feedback from your body is key—listen to it and adapt accordingly.

Incorporating these peptides into your recovery routine not only aids in managing pain and swelling but also supports long-term healing goals. As you navigate through your rehabilitation journey, these peptides offer a promising avenue to enhance recovery outcomes, ensuring you return to your activities stronger and more resilient than before.

Recovery Chronicles: Real-Life Healing Stories

Professional Athletic Recovery

In the dynamic arena of recovery, peptides have become unsung heroes, crafting stories of resilience and triumph. Let's start with a compelling case study: a professional athlete sidelined by a severe knee injury. Conventional treatments offered limited progress, but with the introduction of tailored peptide protocols, the healing process accelerated remarkably. The athlete experienced not only reduced inflammation but also enhanced tissue regeneration, allowing an unexpectedly swift return to competition. Such success stories highlight the transformative power of peptides in sports recovery, where speed and efficacy are paramount.

Chronic Condition Management

Another striking example comes from individuals managing chronic inflammatory conditions. Here, peptides have emerged as a beacon of hope. Consider a patient battling rheumatoid arthritis, a condition notorious for its persistent pain and joint damage. With a personalized peptide regimen, the patient experienced significant reductions in joint swelling and improved mobility. This approach provided relief where traditional therapies fell short, showcasing peptides as a viable alternative in chronic disease management.

Key Success Factors

Analyzing these recovery journeys reveals a common thread: the initial injury assessment and precise peptide selection are critical. Tailoring protocols to individual needs ensures maximum efficacy. As recovery progresses, continuous monitoring and adjustments become essential. This iterative process allows for fine-tuning, ensuring that the body receives exactly what it needs at each stage of healing. It's like steering a ship, making slight course corrections to reach the desired destination safely.

Lessons Learned

Key lessons emerge from these experiences:

- **Personalized protocols** – Not just beneficial but crucial. Each person's unique physiology demands a customized approach

- **Comprehensive monitoring** – Regular check-ins with healthcare professionals and adaptive strategies ensure that peptide therapy aligns with evolving needs, maximizing benefits while minimizing risks

- **Holistic support** – Forms the backbone of successful recovery

Inspirational Outcomes

The inspirational outcomes speak volumes. Personal stories abound with tales of overcoming injury challenges. One individual shared how peptides helped them regain not just physical function but also emotional resilience, enhancing their quality of life post-recovery. Testimonials echo this sentiment, with users expressing gratitude for the renewed vitality and strength peptides bring to their lives.

As we wrap up this chapter, it's clear that peptides have fundamentally changed the landscape of recovery and repair. They offer hope and healing where traditional methods may falter, empowering individuals to reclaim their lives with renewed vigor. Peptide therapy is not one-size-fits-all. Personalized protocols ensure better results and fewer side effects based on individual needs, health goals, and physiological differences [40]. Looking ahead, we'll delve into how peptides play a role in enhancing overall vitality and longevity in our next chapter on extending life through advanced biohacking strategies.

Chapter Ten
Mind Medicine
Peptides and Mental Health

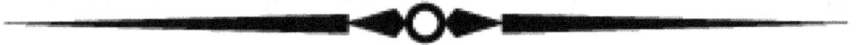

———◀◆O◆▶———

Brain Chemistry: Peptides and Mental Wellness

I magine walking into a room filled with sunlight where your mind feels alive and refreshed. This is what peptides can do for mental health. They offer a new lens through which we can view emotional well-being, working at the junction of brain chemistry and emotional regulation. Peptides interact intimately with neurotransmitter systems, the tiny messengers like serotonin and dopamine that dictate how we think and feel. By influencing these pathways, peptides help maintain a neurochemical balance that supports a stable mood and sharp cognition.

Potential Mental Health Benefits

The potential benefits of peptides for mental health are vast:

- **Anxiety reduction** – They can reduce anxiety symptoms by modulating the release and reception of neurotransmitters, creating a calming effect on the mind

- **Cognitive clarity** – For those dealing with mood disorders, peptides offer cognitive clarity, helping lift the fog that often accompanies such conditions

- **Natural relief** – Imagine struggling with anxiety only to find relief through a natural compound that speaks directly to your brain's chemistry

Scientific Foundation

Scientific research backs these claims, shedding light on how peptides can reshape mental wellness. Studies show that certain peptides enhance neuroplasticity, the brain's ability to adapt and form new connections [49]. This flexibility is crucial in overcoming mental health challenges. Research also highlights peptides' role in treating depression, offering hope through mechanisms that traditional treatments might miss [50]. These findings underscore the promising role of peptides in mental health care.

Integration with Traditional Therapy

In modern therapy, peptides act as valuable allies. They complement traditional approaches like psychotherapy and medication, working alongside them to enhance outcomes. In clinical settings, they serve as adjunctive treatments, providing additional support for those navigating complex emotional landscapes. By integrating peptides into existing mental health strategies, individuals can achieve a more holistic approach to well-being.

Reflection Exercise: Mental Wellness Assessment

Take a moment to reflect on your mental wellness journey. Note any areas where you feel peptides could support your emotional balance or cognitive clarity. Keep this in mind as we explore further applications of peptides in mental health.

Peptides represent a frontier in mental health care, offering tools to enhance emotional resilience and cognitive function. Their ability to work seamlessly with traditional therapies paves the way for more comprehensive care. As we continue to explore these compounds, their role in mental wellness becomes increasingly significant, opening new avenues for those seeking enhanced mental clarity and emotional stability.

Stress Soothers: Peptides for Calm and Balance

How Peptides Combat Stress

Imagine the calm that washes over you when stress melts away, leaving clarity and peace. Peptides play a pivotal role in managing stress by mediating the body's response to stressors and promoting relaxation. These small chains of amino acids have a significant influence on cortisol levels, the hormone that spikes during stress, which can wreak havoc on the body if left unchecked.

By modulating cortisol production, peptides help keep this hormone at healthy levels, preventing it from dictating your mood and energy. Additionally, peptides encourage the activity of the parasympathetic nervous system, which is responsible for rest and digestion. Think of it as the body's natural brake pedal, slowing everything down to restore balance.

Key Stress-Relief Peptides

Several peptides are known for their stress-relief properties:

Selank – Celebrated for its ability to modulate anxiety and provide a sense of calm without sedation. It works by influencing neurotransmitter balance, providing a gentle nudge towards tranquility.

Delta-Sleep-Inducing Peptide (DSIP) – Despite its name, DSIP doesn't just promote sleep; it also enhances relaxation through its calming effects on the central nervous system. This makes it a valuable ally in managing stress, especially when combined with mindfulness practices like meditation.

Implementation Strategies

Incorporating peptides into your stress management routine requires some thought:

Timing and Dosage – Taking Selank in small doses throughout the day can help maintain a steady state of calm, while DSIP might be best used in the evening to prepare for restful sleep.

Synergistic Practices – Pairing peptides with relaxation techniques amplifies their benefits. Practicing mindfulness or engaging in activities like yoga can enhance the calming effects of peptides, creating a holistic approach to stress reduction.

Real-World Success Stories

Real-world stories underscore the effectiveness of peptides in managing stress:

High-Pressure Professionals – Individuals in high-pressure jobs, such as emergency responders or corporate executives, have found relief from chronic stress through peptide use. One executive shared how Selank helped maintain focus and calm during critical business negotiations.

Chronic Stress Conditions – Those with ongoing stress conditions have experienced significant improvements. A teacher dealing with burnout found that DSIP not only improved sleep quality but also provided daytime relief from anxiety.

These testimonials highlight the potential of peptides to transform lives burdened by stress. By integrating these compounds into daily life, you can find a balance that promotes relaxation and mental clarity. Whether you're navigating a high-stress job or dealing with chronic anxiety, peptides offer a promising path to a calmer, more centered existence.

Mood Elevators: Peptides for Emotional Wellbeing

Mechanisms of Mood Regulation

Imagine a day where your emotions remain steady, unshaken by the little things. Peptides can help make this a reality. They work by modulating key neurotransmitter pathways, particularly those involving serotonin and dopamine, which play fundamental roles in mood regulation. By influencing these pathways, peptides can help stabilize mood swings and enhance emotional resilience.

The modulation of serotonin contributes to a sense of well-being and calm, while dopamine affects motivation and pleasure, creating a balanced emotional state that is both resilient and adaptable.

Key Mood-Enhancing Peptides

Among peptides that can enhance mood:

Oxytocin – Stands out for its role in strengthening social bonds and improving mood. Known as the "love hormone," oxytocin fosters feelings of trust and connection, which can be profoundly uplifting. Whether it's a warm hug or a meaningful conversation, oxytocin enhances these experiences, creating a stronger emotional foundation. Research suggests oxytocin may also support emotional wellness in older adults, helping maintain cognitive function and reduce anxiety [51].

Peptide YY (PYY) – Although primarily known for appetite regulation, also contributes to mood stabilization. PYY can help mitigate the emotional highs and lows that often accompany dietary changes or stress.

Scientific Understanding

Delving into the science, peptides influence mood through their regulatory effects on the hypothalamus, a brain region crucial for hormonal balance. By modulating hypothalamic function, peptides help maintain a harmonious balance of hormones that directly impact mood. This regulation facilitates a more stable emotional environment and reduces the impact of stressors on mental well-being. The ability of peptides to fine-tune hormonal responses contributes significantly to their mood-enhancing properties.

Practical Application

When considering mood-enhancing peptides, starting with low doses is wise. This cautious approach allows you to gauge their effects and adjust as needed. It's akin to testing the waters before diving in. Combining peptide use with lifestyle changes—like regular exercise, healthy eating, and mindfulness practices—can amplify their benefits. This holistic strategy supports comprehensive mood enhancement, creating a robust framework for emotional well-being that goes beyond the biochemical.

Incorporating peptides into your daily routine can transform your emotional landscape. Imagine starting your day with the calming influence of oxytocin or ending it with the stabilizing effects of PYY. These small adjustments can make a big difference in how you navigate life's ups and downs. With careful integration and mindful usage, peptides offer a promising path to enhanced emotional resilience and stability.

Mental Health Journeys: Transformative Peptide Stories

Sarah's Anxiety Transformation

Meet Sarah, a young professional who, for years, found herself in the grip of anxiety that turned everyday tasks into monumental challenges. She often felt trapped in her own mind, with a constant hum of worry clouding her days. Through a friend's recommendation, Sarah decided to explore peptides. Under careful guidance, she began incorporating Selank into her routine.

Gradually, the fog lifted. Sarah noticed a newfound clarity and calmness enveloping her. Her racing thoughts slowed, allowing her to engage more fully in her work and personal life. The transformation wasn't overnight, but it was profound. For Sarah, peptides became a cornerstone in regaining control over her mental health.

James's Depression Journey

Then there's James, who faced the heavy burden of depression for much of his adult life. Traditional treatments had provided some relief, but the shadows always lingered. Curious yet cautious, James turned to peptides as an adjunctive therapy. Specifically, he focused on peptides known for their mood-regulating properties.

Over several months, he experienced a subtle yet powerful shift. There was a lightness in his step and an unexpected brightness to his days. James found himself more engaged with his surroundings and more hopeful about his future.

Key Success Factors

These stories highlight an important insight: personalized peptide protocols make a significant difference. Tailoring the dosage and types of peptides to fit individual needs is crucial for maximizing benefits. Consistent use, paired with regular monitoring, ensures that these benefits are sustained over time. It's about finding what works best for your unique chemistry.

Diverse Applications

The diversity of conditions that can benefit from peptides is impressive:

PTSD Recovery – Consider Laura, who faced PTSD after a traumatic event. With guidance, she incorporated peptides into her treatment plan. Over time, she noticed significant improvements in her emotional regulation, allowing her to process experiences with less distress.

Mood Disorders – Think of Mark, who struggled with mood disorders that left him on an emotional rollercoaster. Through careful peptide use, Mark found stability and resilience he hadn't experienced before.

Visual Evidence of Progress

To bring these narratives to life, visual elements like charts or graphs can be incredibly illuminating. Imagine before-and-after mood assessment scores charting Sarah's journey or visual representations of anxiety reduction over time illustrating James's progress. These tools provide tangible evidence of change, making the abstract improvements in mental health more concrete and relatable.

Peptides offer a versatile toolkit for mental health enhancement, supporting individuals across a spectrum of challenges. They provide hope where traditional methods may falter, offering new paths to emotional well-being. In the tapestry of mental health treatments, peptides weave their own unique thread of healing and resilience.

Integrative Approach: Mental Wellness Beyond Peptides

Creating a Comprehensive Framework

Imagine using peptides not just as standalone solutions, but as part of a larger framework for mental wellness. By incorporating them into an integrated mental health plan, you can enhance their effectiveness and realize benefits that extend beyond immediate relief.

Professional Collaboration

Working with mental health professionals becomes crucial here. These experts can help create treatment plans that include peptides as complementary tools.

They understand the nuances of mental health and can tailor protocols that align with your unique needs. Communication is key. Regular discussions with therapists and physicians ensure everyone is on the same page, optimizing your care.

Lifestyle Integration

Beyond peptides, lifestyle factors play a significant role in enhancing mental wellness:

Sleep Optimization – Quality sleep acts as a foundation, allowing peptides to work more effectively by ensuring your body's natural repair mechanisms are in top shape. Techniques such as maintaining a consistent sleep schedule or creating a calming bedtime routine can make a world of difference.

Stress Reduction – Mindfulness practices like meditation or yoga complement peptide use. These practices lower stress levels, providing a fertile ground for peptides to amplify their calming effects, creating a more balanced emotional state.

Interestingly, practices like meditation may naturally regulate neuropeptides like oxytocin and vasopressin, which modulate emotional stability and resilience [52].

Building Your Healthcare Team

In this collaborative care approach, finding knowledgeable healthcare providers is essential. Look for professionals who are not only well-versed in mental health but also familiar with peptides. They can offer insights that bridge both traditional and peptide-based treatments. Effective communication strategies further enhance this collaboration. Be open about your experiences and any changes you notice. This transparency allows providers to adjust your treatment plan dynamically, ensuring it remains aligned with your evolving needs.

Long-Term Optimization

For long-term mental health optimization, consider establishing maintenance protocols that extend beyond peptides:

- **Regular monitoring** – Check-ins with healthcare providers help monitor progress and make necessary adjustments

- **Proactive prevention** – Recognizing triggers and managing them before they escalate

- **Managing setbacks** – Flare-ups are part of the journey, but with a robust framework, they become manageable

- **Lifestyle consistency** – Integrating lifestyle changes and maintaining a consistent routine supports sustained mental wellness

As we conclude this chapter, reflect on the potential of an integrative approach to mental wellness. Peptides offer a powerful tool, but when combined with other strategies, they unlock even greater possibilities for emotional resilience and mental clarity. This synergy not only enhances immediate outcomes but supports long-term well-being. As we move forward, consider how these insights can apply to other areas of health and vitality, continuing our exploration into unlocking the full potential of biohacking for a healthier life.

Chapter Eleven

Wellness Integration

Creating Your Peptide Protocol

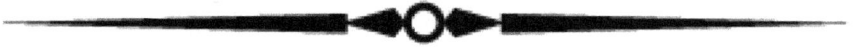

Personalized Planning: Creating Your Peptide Strategy

I magine unlocking a treasure chest filled with health potential—this is what crafting your personalized peptide strategy can offer. At the heart of this journey is a thorough self-assessment, a crucial step in identifying your wellness goals and how peptides can aid you.

Self-Assessment Foundation

Start by completing a wellness questionnaire, examining your current health status, lifestyle habits, and specific challenges you wish to address. Are you looking to boost muscle strength, enhance cognitive function, or improve sleep quality? Pinpoint these goals to steer your peptide choices effectively.

Customization Strategies

Customization is where the magic happens. Tailoring peptide use to fit your health profile amplifies benefits and ensures safe practice. Personalized dosing schedules can help you achieve precise results, just like a well-calibrated watch keeps perfect time. Consider genetic predispositions that may influence how you respond to certain peptides. For example, if you have a family history of metabolic issues, you might focus on peptides known for supporting insulin sensitivity and metabolism. This individualized approach empowers you to optimize your health journey.

Building Your Plan

To build your peptide plan, follow a structured process:

1. **Set specific, measurable goals** – Instead of vague objectives like "feel better," aim for quantifiable targets such as "increase muscle mass by 10% in six months"

2. **Schedule regular progress reviews** – Assess your progress every few weeks, making tweaks as necessary

3. **Embrace iterative improvement** – This process is essential for fine-tuning your regimen and achieving desired outcomes

Professional Guidance

Incorporating professional guidance into your plan is non-negotiable. Collaborate with a peptide specialist who understands the nuances of these compounds. They can provide insights that you might miss and ensure that your protocol is both effective and safe. Leverage technology for health monitoring, using apps and devices to track vital signs and health markers in real-time. These tools offer valuable feedback, helping you make informed decisions about your peptide use.

Interactive Element: Personalized Peptide Plan Checklist

Create a checklist to guide your strategy development. Include items such as setting health goals, selecting peptides, planning dosing schedules, scheduling reviews, and consulting professionals. Use this checklist as a roadmap to navigate your peptide journey with confidence.

By weaving these elements together, you create a robust framework for integrating peptides into your wellness strategy. This personalized approach not only enhances the effectiveness of peptides but also aligns with your unique health needs and aspirations, setting the stage for long-term vitality and well-being.

Nutritional Synergy: Peptides and Diet Working Together

Understanding the Connection

Understanding how peptides and nutrition dance together can be a game-changer. Your diet profoundly impacts peptide efficacy, and likewise, peptides can enhance how your body uses nutrients. Macro and micronutrients play pivotal roles in this equation. Proteins, fats, and carbs fuel bodily functions, while vitamins and minerals fine-tune these processes. A balanced diet ensures that peptides are absorbed and utilized effectively, making the most of their potential.

Synergistic Combinations

Certain peptides thrive when paired with specific dietary practices:

Collagen Peptides – Find an ally in vitamin C-rich foods like oranges and strawberries, which aid in collagen synthesis. This combination supports skin elasticity and joint health.

Nutrient Uptake Peptides – Boost the body's ability to absorb essential vitamins and minerals. Pairing these with a nutrient-dense diet maximizes their benefits.

Dietary Recommendations

Dietary recommendations for peptide users hinge on choosing foods that support overall health while enhancing peptide function:

- **Anti-inflammatory foods** such as fatty fish, berries, and leafy greens complement peptides by reducing bodily inflammation, allowing them to work more efficiently

- **Proper hydration** is another key factor. Water facilitates nutrient transport and aids in peptide metabolism, ensuring they reach their intended targets within the body

Nutrient Timing Strategies

Nutrient timing is another layer to consider. Timing meals can significantly influence peptide effectiveness:

- **Pre and post-workout nutrition** – Consuming a protein-rich meal before and after workouts can bolster amino acid availability, crucial for muscle repair and growth when using peptides aimed at muscle enhancement

- **Absorption optimization** – Aligning meal times with peptide administration can optimize absorption. Taking peptides on an empty stomach might speed up their action, while pairing them with food could slow down digestion, providing a more sustained release

Interactive Element: Meal Timing Planner

Create a chart to visualize your peptide schedule alongside meal times. This planner can help you optimize your dietary practices to complement your peptide regimen, ensuring you make the most of both.

In weaving these nutritional strategies with peptide use, you're setting the stage for enhanced vitality and wellness. These thoughtful combinations not only support your health goals but also elevate the impact of peptides in your daily life. Whether you're focused on building muscle, improving skin health, or boosting cognitive function, integrating diet with peptide use is a powerful approach that amplifies results.

Exercise Enhancement: Maximizing Workout Results with Peptides

The Peptide Advantage in Fitness

In the gym, peptides are like secret weapons, quietly working their magic behind the scenes. They enhance recovery after a workout by accelerating the repair of muscle fibers. This means less soreness and quicker return to peak performance. For those focused on muscle growth, peptides stimulate protein synthesis, which is crucial for building strength. It's like adding fuel to a fire, intensifying the body's natural processes. Imagine finishing a challenging session and feeling ready to tackle the next day with minimal downtime. That's the peptide effect in action.

Goal-Specific Peptide Selection

Different fitness goals call for different peptides:

Endurance Athletes – Peptides like AICAR can boost stamina by enhancing the body's ability to burn fat and improve oxygen delivery. This means longer runs and less fatigue.

Muscle Building – Peptides such as IGF-1 LR3 are your allies. They promote muscle hypertrophy, helping you pack on lean mass efficiently.

Each peptide aligns with specific objectives, making it important to select the right one for your needs.

Timing and Dosage Strategies

Timing and dosage are critical:

Pre-Workout Protocol – Consider peptides designed to prepare your body for exertion. These can improve blood flow and energy levels, giving you an edge as you start your routine.

Post-Workout Recovery – Focus shifts to recovery strategies. Post-workout peptides facilitate muscle repair and reduce inflammation, setting the stage for optimal recovery.

Synchronizing peptide use with your exercise schedule maximizes benefits and enhances performance.

The Exercise-Peptide Synergy

There's a fascinating feedback loop between exercise and peptides. Regular physical activity boosts circulation, which in turn improves peptide delivery throughout the body. When you exercise, you also experience hormonal changes that can amplify peptide activity, creating a synergistic effect. This interplay accelerates your progress, as each element—exercise and peptides—enhances the other's effectiveness. The result is a cycle of continuous improvement.

Interactive Element: Peptide-Exercise Logbook

Consider keeping a logbook where you record your workouts alongside your peptide use. Note changes in energy levels, recovery time, and performance metrics. This log will allow you to track how effectively your peptide regimen complements your exercise routine.

Incorporating peptides into your fitness regimen isn't just about taking supplements; it's about creating a comprehensive strategy that aligns with your physical goals. By understanding how to integrate these powerful compounds with your workouts, you unlock new levels of strength and endurance.

Progress Tracking: Measuring Your Peptide Success

The Importance of Monitoring

Tracking your progress when using peptides is like having a compass on a foggy day—it guides you and keeps your path clear. By regularly monitoring your progress, you can determine whether your peptide protocol is effective or needs tweaking. Patterns in performance and trends in results become apparent over time, offering valuable insights.

Perhaps you notice that your energy levels peak a day after peptide administration or that muscle recovery accelerates with specific dosages. By identifying these trends, you can make informed adjustments to your regimen, ensuring that each dose maximizes your potential.

Technology Tools

In today's tech-savvy world, various tools can help you keep track of your progress:

Wearable Fitness Trackers – Provide real-time data on heart rate, sleep patterns, and activity levels. Wearable tech like fitness trackers can help monitor HRV, sleep, and activity, which are all impacted by peptide protocols [53].These gadgets offer a window into how your body responds to peptides, allowing for precise adjustments.

Nutrition Apps – Take on the task of logging dietary intake, ensuring that your nutritional habits align with your peptide goals.

Blood Tests – Though more involved, provide crucial biomarker analysis that can reveal how peptides influence your internal physiology.

Together, these tools create a comprehensive picture of your health journey.

Data Interpretation

Understanding the data you collect is crucial. Setting measurable goals and benchmarks makes interpreting your progress straightforward. Are you aiming to increase muscle mass by a certain percentage? Or perhaps you're looking to improve sleep quality? By setting these clear objectives, you can use the collected data to fine-tune your peptide and exercise protocols.

A spike in energy levels might suggest an adjustment in timing, while consistent fatigue could indicate a need for dosage modification. Data-driven insights transform guesswork into a strategic approach.

Success Stories

Consider the stories of athletes who have successfully harnessed the power of monitoring to optimize their strategies:

The Strategic Runner – One runner used wearable data to identify their peak performance times, aligning peptide use accordingly to enhance stamina during races.

The Nutrition-Focused Athlete – Another athlete tracked dietary intake alongside peptides, discovering that certain foods significantly boosted energy post-workout.

Graphs and charts vividly illustrate these journeys, showing tangible progress over time. They provide not just motivation but also concrete evidence of what works.

Visual Element: Progress Graphs and Charts

Visualize your peptide journey through graphs and charts. Map out your progress over weeks or months, noting changes in performance metrics. This visual representation offers clarity and motivation, helping you see where you've been and where you're heading.

Monitoring and tracking form the backbone of successful peptide use. They empower you to make informed decisions, leading to more effective protocols and better results. By embracing these tools and techniques, you're not just supplementing with peptides; you're transforming how you engage with health and wellness.

Mind-Body Balance: Mindfulness and Peptide Optimization

The Power of the Mind-Body Connection

In the pursuit of wellness, the mind-body connection is a powerful tool. Mindfulness practices can significantly enhance the effects of peptides, serving as the glue that binds together the physical and mental aspects of health optimization. When stress is reduced, peptides work more effectively, as the body is in a state of balance and receptivity.

Stress can act as a barrier, obstructing the pathways through which peptides exert their benefits. By adopting mindfulness, you create an environment where peptides can perform optimally, enhancing your journey to health.

Mindfulness Techniques

Mindfulness techniques offer a range of practices that complement peptide use:

Meditation – A cornerstone of stress management. It calms the mind and reduces cortisol levels, a hormone that can interfere with peptide function. By incorporating meditation into your routine, you create a peaceful mental landscape where peptides can thrive.

Breathing Exercises – Another powerful ally. They improve mental clarity and focus, allowing you to engage with your wellness journey more fully. These practices don't just support peptide effectiveness; they enrich your mental and emotional well-being.

Psychological Benefits

The psychological benefits of combining mindfulness with peptides are profound:

- **Reduced anxiety and improved mood** are common experiences among those who practice both

- **Mental reset** – Mindfulness helps reset the mind, providing a fresh perspective on challenges and emotions

- **Enhanced focus** – Mindfulness sharpens your mental acuity, making you more present and aware

It's like hitting the reset button on your mental state, allowing peptides to work without the hindrance of stress-induced barriers.

Holistic Integration

Adopting a holistic wellness approach means integrating these practices into a broader health strategy. It's about cultivating a balanced lifestyle that nurtures both body and mind. A proactive approach to personal wellness involves embracing a variety of strategies, from diet and exercise to mindfulness and peptide use. Each element enhances the others, creating a synergy that amplifies overall health benefits. This comprehensive approach ensures that every aspect of your life supports your wellness goals.

In essence, mindfulness is not just an addition to your routine but an integral part of optimizing peptide effectiveness. By embracing these practices, you pave a smooth path for peptides to work their magic, enhancing your health in ways that go beyond the physical.

As we conclude this chapter, remember that wellness is a tapestry woven from many threads—each practice strengthens the whole. In our next chapter, we'll explore how peptides play a role in crafting a life filled with vitality and longevity, continuing this exploration into holistic health. Stay tuned for insights on how to integrate these powerful tools into every aspect of your life, ensuring that you're not just living but thriving.

Chapter Twelve

Safety Shield

Addressing Concerns and Misconceptions

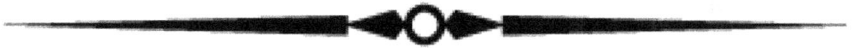

Myth Busters: Debunking Common Peptide Misconceptions

When I first started exploring peptides, I encountered a surprising amount of misinformation that clouded the truth. It's like navigating a maze where myths lurk around every corner.

Common Myths vs. Reality

Myth: Peptides are like anabolic steroids One of the most persistent myths is that peptides are akin to anabolic steroids, leading many to believe they are illegal or dangerous. This misconception stems from their association with muscle growth. Unlike steroids, peptides are chains of amino acids that naturally occur in the body and function differently. They don't alter your hormonal balance in the way steroids do. Instead, they support cellular processes, enhancing your body's natural capabilities.

Myth: Peptides are only for bodybuilders The notion that peptides are only for bodybuilders is another common myth. While athletes do use them to aid recovery and performance, their benefits extend far beyond the gym. Peptides play roles in skin health, cognitive function, and even sleep improvement, making them versatile tools for anyone seeking better health.

Legal Classification and Regulation

Understanding the legality of peptides is crucial. In the U.S., peptides are classified based on their intended use. Many peptides are perfectly legal when used for medical purposes, falling under FDA regulations. They have therapeutic applications approved for certain conditions, distinguishing them from controlled substances like steroids. For instance, oxytocin is used in medicine to manage childbirth and mental health (Lanctot, n.d.). Regulatory bodies ensure that medically approved peptides adhere to strict safety standards, providing reassurance about their legitimacy.

Scientific Evidence

Scientific research supports the efficacy and safety of peptides, dispelling myths with evidence. Studies show that peptides contribute to cellular health by aiding in processes like cell signaling and repair (Peptide Society, n.d.). For example, collagen peptides have been shown to improve skin elasticity and reduce signs of aging, backed by clinical trials (Medical News Today, n.d.). Such evidence highlights how peptides enhance well-being when used correctly, offering benefits grounded in science rather than speculation.

Expert Perspectives

Expert insights further clarify peptide misconceptions. Endocrinologists and peptide specialists emphasize the importance of understanding peptide functions and correct usage. They stress that when sourced responsibly and used according to guidelines, peptides can be safe and effective. Regulatory bodies like the FDA provide statements on peptide safety, underscoring their role in approved medical treatments (Rupa Health, n.d.).

Case Study: Expert Insight on Peptide Legitimacy

Dr. Michael Aziz, a peptide therapy specialist in New York, shares his perspective on peptide safety (Dr. Michael Aziz, n.d.). He notes that when patients follow recommended protocols and consult professionals, they experience significant health improvements without adverse effects. His practice exemplifies the responsible use of peptides in therapeutic settings, reinforcing their potential as valuable health tools.

By dispelling myths and providing clarity, we create a foundation for informed decisions about peptide use. Understanding peptides' true nature allows you to appreciate their potential benefits without fear or misinformation clouding your judgment.

Side Effect Spotlight: What to Watch For

Understanding Potential Reactions

In our quest for improved health, it's crucial to understand potential side effects that may accompany peptide use. Awareness is your first line of defense.

Common Side Effects

Injection Site Reactions Some users report skin reactions at injection sites like redness or swelling. These typically occur when the body reacts to the injection itself rather than the peptide. It's much like when you get a mosquito bite—annoying but usually harmless.

Hormonal Fluctuations Hormonal fluctuations can also arise, though they are less common. Peptides that influence hormone levels might cause imbalances, leading to mood swings or fatigue.

Digestive Disturbances Digestive disturbances, such as nausea or bloating, are rare but possible, usually linked to peptides that impact metabolic processes.

Frequency and Severity

The frequency and severity of these side effects vary. Clinical trials suggest that mild reactions are more common than severe ones, akin to the occasional headache from too much screen time. Most are manageable and diminish as your body adjusts. According to statistics, skin reactions are the most reported, with hormonal imbalances and digestive issues trailing behind (Medical News Today, n.d.). Severe reactions are rare and often linked to incorrect dosing or improper administration, highlighting the importance of following guidelines.

Monitoring and Management

Symptom Tracking Monitoring your body's responses is vital. Keeping a symptom diary can help track any changes you notice, offering valuable insights into what your body is experiencing.

Professional Oversight Regular check-ups with healthcare providers ensure that any potential issues are caught early. These professionals can provide tailored advice, adjusting protocols as needed to maintain your health and safety. Imagine having a trusted guide by your side, ensuring you're on the right path.

Risk Minimization Strategies

To minimize risks, proper injection techniques are pivotal:

- Sterilize equipment thoroughly and ensure the injection site is clean, much like when a chef preps ingredients before cooking

- Gradually adjusting dosages allows your body to acclimate without overwhelming it

- This slow and steady approach reduces the likelihood of adverse reactions

- Think of it as easing into a new exercise routine—start small and build up gradually

Visual Element: Symptom Diary Template

Create a simple template for tracking any side effects or changes in well-being. Include sections for date, symptom description, severity, duration, and any actions taken. This tool aids in identifying patterns and informs discussions with healthcare providers.

Understanding these aspects helps you navigate peptide use wisely. By staying informed and vigilant, you reduce risks while maximizing benefits. Peptides can be powerful allies in achieving your health goals when used responsibly.

Safety Protocols: Essential Guidelines for Protection

Fundamental Preparation

In the intricate world of peptides, ensuring one's safety is paramount. Mastering the fundamental guidelines becomes indispensable for anyone embarking on this journey.

Sterilization and Hygiene

Begin by understanding the importance of thorough preparation before using peptides. Sterilization isn't merely a casual suggestion—it's an imperative action that underscores the importance of hygiene. Picture this as your primary shield against unwanted complications.

Each time you prepare for an injection, ensuring your equipment is pristine is non-negotiable:

- Utilize alcohol swabs diligently to sanitize both the intended skin area and the needle

- Think of it akin to a surgeon meticulously preparing for a procedure

- This simple yet crucial act serves as a barrier, significantly reducing the risk of infections

Proper Storage Practices

Proper storage practices cannot be understated. Peptides require careful attention much like sensitive produce that spoils without adequate preservation:

- Store them in a cool, dark environment—ideally in a refrigerator

- This maintains their efficacy and prolongs their lifespan

Healthcare Professional Integration

Incorporating the expertise of healthcare professionals into your peptide plan is akin to setting a reliable compass for your journey. Consistent medical consultations act as a safety net, offering the peace of mind needed to tailor your regimen effectively. Working with a knowledgeable practitioner ensures safer and more targeted peptide use tailored to your health status [54].

Healthcare experts bring a wealth of knowledge, often identifying nuances that might be easy to miss, ensuring that your dosage is aligned perfectly with your body's unique requirements. In instances where unusual symptoms crop up, these professionals serve as a reassuring resource, ready to provide guidance and modify your approach as necessary. Envision them as co-pilots in your expedition, armed with the acumen to navigate potential hazards adeptly.

Quality Sourcing

When acquiring peptides, prioritizing quality is absolutely critical. The market is teeming with numerous options, making the ability to discern trustworthy suppliers an invaluable skill:

- Seek out brands that demonstrate transparency in their processes and submit to rigorous third-party testing

- Be wary of those that make grandiose claims which seem implausibly beneficial

- Equip yourself with ample information—customer reviews and obtaining certifications are indispensable allies

- Buyers should look for third-party testing, purity certificates, and vendor transparency when sourcing peptides online [55]

Knowledge and Education

In understanding peptides and making informed decisions, knowledge indeed equates to empowerment. Immerse yourself in scientific literature and reputable resources to illuminate the path forward. This doesn't entail becoming an overnight scientist but grasping the foundational elements that lead to informed decision-making. Engaging with support groups or online forums can provide you with invaluable, pragmatic insights from individuals traversing similar paths, allowing their experiences to seamlessly transform into your learning moments.

Approaching peptide usage with a comprehensive and thorough strategy not only fortifies your health but also maximizes the potential benefits available. Similar to any sophisticated tool, peptides offer the most value when employed responsibly and with precision. Regard this as your comprehensive blueprint for success, where each deliberate step underscores a dedication to both safety and efficacy.

Special Considerations: Who Should Exercise Caution

High-Risk Populations

Peptides can be powerful allies in achieving specific health goals, but it's crucial to recognize that certain individuals should approach them with caution or even avoid them entirely.

Pregnancy and Nursing

Pregnant and nursing mothers are advised to steer clear of peptide use. During these sensitive periods, the body's hormonal landscape is already in flux, and introducing peptides could potentially disrupt delicate balances, posing risks to both mother and child.

Cancer Patients

Cancer patients should exercise caution. Some peptides might stimulate cell growth, which could inadvertently accelerate tumor progression. It's essential for these individuals to consult their healthcare provider before considering peptide therapy.

Specific Medical Conditions

Those with specific medical conditions also need to tread carefully:

Autoimmune Disorders – Present unique challenges. Peptides that modulate the immune system might exacerbate symptoms in individuals with conditions like lupus or rheumatoid arthritis.

Endocrine Issues – Such as thyroid disorders or adrenal insufficiency, peptides that influence hormonal pathways could complicate their condition.

This makes it vital for anyone with existing health concerns to engage in detailed discussions with their doctor before starting peptide use.

Medication Interactions

Medication interactions are another critical aspect to consider:

Anticoagulants – Which thin the blood to prevent clots, might interact unfavorably with certain peptides that influence platelet activity or coagulation pathways. This could increase bleeding risk.

Hormone Therapy – Those undergoing hormone therapy should be aware of potential interactions with peptides that affect hormonal balance. These interactions might alter the effectiveness of their current treatment plan, leading to unintended consequences.

Reproductive Health Considerations

For individuals concerned about reproductive health, awareness is key. While research is ongoing, some peptides could influence fertility by altering hormonal levels or reproductive organ function. It's wise to approach peptide use cautiously if you're planning a family or concerned about fertility. Additionally, the developmental risks for unborn children remain largely unexplored, underscoring the need for restraint during pregnancy.

Age-Related Considerations

Age plays a significant role in how peptides affect the body:

Adolescents – Whose bodies are still developing, may experience altered growth patterns if they engage in peptide use. The potential impact on growth plates and hormonal development necessitates a conservative approach for this age group.

Older Adults – Might face different challenges. As metabolism slows with age, the way peptides are processed and utilized can change. This might require adjusting dosages to ensure safety and effectiveness without overburdening the body's systems.

In these cases, personalized guidance from a healthcare professional can make all the difference. They can help tailor peptide regimens to individual needs, ensuring that any risks are minimized while maximizing potential benefits. It's about finding that balance—using peptides strategically to enhance well-being without compromising health.

Evidence-Based Confidence: Addressing Peptide Skepticism

Understanding Natural Skepticism

Skepticism towards peptides is understandable, especially in a world where new therapies often emerge faster than the research to back them up. Many folks worry about diving into unfamiliar waters, fearing unproven methods without a clear track record. Concerns about long-term safety and efficacy loom large; after all, you want to be sure that what you're introducing into your body will benefit you without hidden drawbacks. This apprehension is not only natural but healthy, prompting us to seek reassurance.

Scientific Foundation

Fortunately, science provides a comforting hand. Numerous studies and data reinforce the positive impact of peptides. Case studies abound with success stories—patients with chronic conditions finding relief and improved quality of life through peptide therapy. For instance, meta-analyses indicate substantial improvements in muscle recovery and skin health, painting a picture of peptides as allies rather than adversaries. This scientific backing helps alleviate fears, offering a foundation of trust built on evidence.

Regulatory Legitimacy

Legitimacy shines through in the regulatory approvals peptides have secured. The FDA has given the nod to various peptide therapies for specific medical uses, underscoring their safety and effectiveness. Peptides like insulin have been transformative in managing diabetes, while others are approved for growth deficiencies and hormone regulation. These endorsements reflect rigorous scrutiny, ensuring that only well-substantiated therapies make the cut. International regulatory bodies echo these approvals, further solidifying confidence in peptide applications.

Personal Success Stories

Personal stories often resonate deeply, offering relatable insights that data alone may not convey. Patients who've battled chronic ailments share their triumphs, attributing newfound vitality to peptides. Take athletes who've leveraged peptides to enhance recovery times and performance levels—these testimonials highlight tangible benefits difficult to ignore. They serve as beacons of hope, illustrating the real-world impact of peptides in diverse contexts.

Textual Element: Testimonial Collection

Consider the experiences of individuals who have embraced peptides with transformative results:

Jane's Story – A middle-aged professional, credits peptide therapy for her renewed energy and resilience against autoimmune challenges.

Mark's Achievement – An athlete, shares how peptides shaved precious seconds off his race times, elevating his competitive edge.

These narratives provide not just inspiration but validation for those contemplating similar paths.

In wrapping up this chapter, we see how evidence dispels skepticism and builds bridges of understanding. Peptides, when approached with informed caution and scientific backing, emerge as remarkable tools in our health arsenal. As we move forward, the focus will shift to integrating these insights into actionable strategies for holistic wellness and vitality in the next chapter—because health is more than just the absence of illness; it's about thriving at every level.

Chapter Thirteen

Problem Solving

Troubleshooting Common Issues

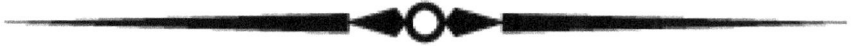

———◆○◆———

Results Refinement: Managing Inconsistent Outcomes

I magine setting out on a journey only to find the path unexpectedly winding and uneven. This can feel similar to navigating the world of peptides when results fluctuate. These inconsistencies often stem from individual variations—our genetics play a crucial role. Just like how some people metabolize caffeine differently, peptides interact with our unique genetic makeup in varied ways. This can lead to different outcomes in terms of effectiveness.

Common Causes of Inconsistency

Individual Genetic Variations:

Our genetics play a crucial role in how peptides work for us. Just like some people metabolize caffeine differently, peptides interact with our unique genetic makeup in varied ways, leading to different outcomes in terms of effectiveness.

Incorrect Dosing

Another common culprit is incorrect dosing. If you don't administer peptides at the right time or in the correct amount, you might experience less-than-ideal results. Timing is everything, and a misstep here can throw a wrench into your peptide plans.

Strategies for Consistency

To smooth out these fluctuations, begin by maintaining a consistent administration schedule. Regularity helps your body adapt, reducing variability:

Detailed Tracking Keep a detailed log of your peptide use and observed outcomes. This tracking not only provides insight into what works but also highlights patterns that might need addressing.

Protocol Adjustments Adjusting protocols based on these insights is key. If a certain dosage isn't yielding the desired effect, modify it slightly and observe any changes.

Administration Methods Experimenting with different administration routes might also reveal unforeseen benefits. Your body might respond better to one method over another, unlocking greater potential.

When to Seek Professional Help

But sometimes, despite our best efforts, inconsistencies persist. That's when consulting professionals becomes invaluable:

- **Healthcare providers** offer personalized guidance, honing in on what might be going awry

- **Peptide specialists** bring a wealth of expertise to your side

- **Professional assessment** can suggest adjustments that align better with your unique physiology

- **Expert insight** transforms guesswork into informed action, steering you towards reliable results

Interactive Element: Consultation Checklist

Create a checklist for your next consultation with healthcare providers or peptide specialists. List questions about dosing, administration methods, and potential adjustments based on your observed outcomes. This preparation ensures you maximize the value of your professional consultations and move closer to consistent, effective peptide use.

Navigating these challenges is part of the journey—each step refines your approach, bringing you closer to unlocking the full potential of peptides.

Side Effect Solutions: Addressing Unexpected Reactions

When venturing into peptide use, unexpected reactions can sometimes crop up, throwing a wrench into your plans for self-improvement.

Managing Common Side Effects

Injection Site Irritation Common side effects might include irritation at the injection site. This could feel like a mild itch or redness. Managing such irritation can often be as simple as applying a soothing topical treatment—think aloe vera or a gentle hydrocortisone cream. These can calm the skin, reducing discomfort.

Mild Flu-Like Symptoms You might experience mild flu-like symptoms; rest and hydration can be your best allies here. Take it easy for a day or two, ensuring you drink plenty of fluids to help your body adjust.

Recognizing Serious Reactions

It's crucial to stay alert for more severe reactions:

Allergic Reactions Symptoms like hives or difficulty breathing could indicate an allergic reaction. These are red flags requiring immediate attention.

Systemic Issues Persistent headaches or dizziness might suggest systemic issues. While they may seem minor at first, they can signal underlying problems needing professional evaluation.

Regularly monitor how your body responds to peptides, noting any significant changes or persistent discomforts.

Prevention Strategies

To minimize side effects, focus on proper protocols from the get-go:

- **Proper injection technique** can make a big difference

- **Use clean, sterile equipment** and practice good hygiene to prevent infections

- **Start with low dosage** and gradually increase to allow your body to adjust without overwhelming it

When to Seek Medical Intervention

Knowing when to seek medical intervention is vital:

- If side effects **persist or worsen**, don't hesitate to contact a healthcare provider

- **New or unusual symptoms** that weren't previously experienced should also prompt a visit to your doctor

- Healthcare providers can offer guidance and potentially adjust your regimen to better suit your needs

Visual Element: Symptom Diary Template

Consider keeping a symptom diary. Jot down any reactions you notice after taking peptides—both the mild and the more intense ones. This practice helps track patterns and provides valuable information for healthcare consultations. It aids in pinpointing triggers and adjusting your approach for improved safety and effectiveness.

Managing side effects with peptides doesn't have to be daunting. By staying informed and proactive, you can enjoy the benefits while minimizing risks.

Quality Control: Identifying and Avoiding Fake Products

In the realm of peptides, ensuring you get what you pay for can sometimes resemble a game of detective work. Counterfeit products lurk in the market, and their signs can be subtle yet telling.

Red Flags to Watch For

Packaging Inconsistencies One of the most glaring indicators is inconsistent labeling or packaging discrepancies. If you notice packaging that seems off—perhaps labels that don't align properly or text in an unusual font—it's wise to question the product's authenticity.

Suspiciously Low Pricing Suspiciously low pricing is another red flag. While we all love a good deal, remember that if it seems too good to be true, it probably is. Unverified sources offering rock-bottom prices are often peddling inferior or fake peptides, which can pose serious health risks.

Verification Steps

Before making any purchase, take steps to verify product authenticity:
Third-Party Testing Look for third-party testing or certification. Legiti-

mate suppliers will often provide evidence of their products' purity and efficacy through independent lab results.

Supplier Research Spend some time researching the reputation of the supplier or manufacturer. Established companies usually have a track record of positive reviews and transparent practices. Peptide Society (2023) highlights the importance of understanding the science behind peptides to make informed decisions and verify authenticity (Peptide Society, n.d.).

Best Purchasing Practices

When it comes to purchasing peptides, best practices can shield you from counterfeit pitfalls:

- **Always buy from reputable, well-reviewed vendors** who have built trust within the community

- **Avoid online marketplaces without verification processes**—these platforms can be breeding grounds for counterfeit goods

- **Seek vendors who prioritize customer education** and transparency in their sourcing and manufacturing processes

Responding to Counterfeit Products

If you do find yourself with a counterfeit product, knowing how to respond is crucial:

Report to Authorities Reporting it to relevant regulatory authorities helps protect others from similar experiences. These agencies can investigate and take action against fraudulent suppliers, cleaning up the market for everyone.

Community Awareness Additionally, sharing your experience in online communities can warn fellow peptide enthusiasts. Your insights can help others avoid the same pitfalls and encourage vigilance within the community.

The peptide landscape is filled with potential, yet navigating it requires discernment. By staying informed and proactive, you can enjoy the benefits of peptides while minimizing risks associated with counterfeit products.

Plateau Breakers: Overcoming Stalled Progress

Hitting a plateau can feel like driving at full speed, only to hit a roadblock you can't quite see. This happens often with peptide use, and understanding why is crucial.

Understanding Plateaus

Tolerance Development One of the main reasons is the development of tolerance. Over time, your body may adapt to the peptides, reducing their effectiveness. It's as if your body starts ignoring the signals it once responded to eagerly.

Lifestyle Factors Another factor is the lack of complementary lifestyle adjustments. Peptides work best when paired with a healthy lifestyle. If you're not adjusting your diet, exercise, or sleep patterns, you might be stalling their potential benefits.

Breakthrough Strategies

Breaking through these plateaus requires a bit of strategy:

Cycling Protocols Implementing cycling protocols can help reset your body's response. By taking planned breaks from peptides, you allow your body to recalibrate its sensitivity to them. Think of it like rebooting a sluggish computer—it gives everything a fresh start.

Peptide Combinations Introducing complementary peptides can also create synergy, enhancing overall efficacy. Each peptide has strengths, and strategically combining them can lead to better results than using one alone.

Dosage Fine-Tuning Fine-tuning dosages is another way to overcome stagnation. Sometimes a small adjustment can reignite progress. It's about finding that sweet spot where the peptide is most effective for you.

New Combinations Experimenting with new peptide combinations can also uncover new pathways to progress. Different peptides interact uniquely, and you may find that a new combination offers just the boost you need.

Monitoring and Feedback

Constant monitoring and feedback are vital in this process:

Goal Setting Setting new performance or health goals keeps your motivation alive and provides benchmarks to measure progress against.

Data Tracking Utilizing biomarkers and data tracking offers concrete insights into how your body is responding. These metrics guide your decisions, ensuring adjustments are informed rather than guesswork.

Textual Element: Peptide Adjustment Journal

Consider keeping a journal dedicated to tracking your peptide use, lifestyle changes, and any progress or setbacks. This log becomes a powerful tool in identifying patterns and making informed adjustments. Note any changes in energy levels, muscle gain, or recovery times alongside detailed descriptions of your peptide regimen. This practice not only helps you identify what's working but also highlights areas for improvement.

Adjustments in peptide use aren't just about dosage tweaks or adding new compounds; they reflect a broader commitment to achieving your health goals. By understanding the factors at play and actively engaging with these strategies, you position yourself to break through plateaus and unlock new levels of wellness.

Decision Guide: Problem-Solving Flowcharts

Navigating the world of peptides can sometimes feel like solving a complex puzzle. With so many moving parts, creating a systematic approach to diagnosing and resolving issues becomes crucial.

Diagnostic Approach

Progressive Symptom Assessment Imagine having a diagnostic flowchart at your disposal, a tool designed to streamline the process of identifying peptide-related problems. Start with a progressive symptom assessment, examining any signs your body presents and noting any inconsistencies. From mild discomfort to more pronounced symptoms, each clue plays a role in narrowing down potential causes. This methodology helps pinpoint issues with precision, reducing guesswork and allowing you to focus on the most likely culprits.

Resolution Framework

Step-by-Step Solutions Once you have a clearer picture of the problem, a step-by-step resolution guide becomes your best ally:

1. **Administration Technique Adjustments** – Small tweaks, like altering injection angles or locations, can make significant differences in outcomes

2. **Dosage Modifications** – Sometimes, even minor adjustments can lead to substantial improvements, aligning your protocols with your body's unique needs

3. **Protocol Refinement** – This structured approach provides clarity and direction, transforming challenges into manageable tasks

Decision Criteria

Adjust vs. Discontinue Deciding whether to adjust or discontinue peptide use requires clear criteria:

Minor Side Effects – Can often be managed with simple techniques, such as topical treatments for irritation

Serious Adverse Reactions – Demand immediate attention and potential discontinuation

Understanding these distinctions is crucial for maintaining safety while optimizing benefits. This decision-making process empowers you to act confidently, knowing when to push forward and when to pull back.

Preventative Strategies

Maintenance Best Practices Preventative maintenance strategies play a vital role in avoiding common issues altogether:

Proper Storage and Handling – Ensure peptides retain their effectiveness over time. Keep them cool and dry, safeguarding them from environmental degradation.

Quality Verification – By sourcing peptides from reputable suppliers and verifying their authenticity, you minimize the risk of encountering subpar products.

These proactive steps create a solid foundation for success, reducing the likelihood of encountering problems.

As we wrap up this chapter on troubleshooting common peptide issues, remember that each challenge is an opportunity for growth and refinement. By equipping yourself with the right tools and knowledge, you transform potential roadblocks into stepping stones, paving the way for more effective and satisfying peptide use. The following chapter will delve into optimizing your peptide experience even further, exploring advanced strategies for enhancing performance and vitality. Stay tuned as we continue this journey into the fascinating world of peptides, unlocking new potential at every turn.

Chapter Fourteen
Future Horizons
Emerging Peptide Research

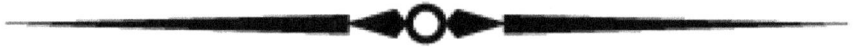

Research Frontiers: Breakthrough Peptide Discoveries

Envision a world where the tiniest fragments of proteins, intriguingly termed peptides, act as the driving force behind groundbreaking medical advancements. This is no mere figment of fantasy but stands as the forefront of scientific progression today. In recent years, peptide research has boldly traversed into previously unknown territories, paving the way for thrilling new applications.

Novel Peptide Sequences

Researchers have unveiled a multitude of novel peptide sequences, each harboring unique functions that defy conventional biological wisdom. These sequences are far more than arbitrary chains; they represent meticulously structured molecules, deliberately designed to interact intricately with biological systems in unprecedented ways, thus revolutionizing conventional medical paradigms.

Their synthesis and stability have undergone tremendous enhancements, addressing and resolving challenges that had once hindered their widespread adoption in medical practices [56]. Through these advancements, peptides have proven themselves to be not only viable candidates but also superior options for therapeutic interventions.

Regenerative Medicine Applications

In the realm of regenerative medicine, peptides are diligently sculpting a niche for themselves. By adeptly mimicking the body's intrinsic healing mechanisms, they present a beacon of hope for the restoration of damaged tissues and organs. Acting as a biological scaffold, these peptides guide and facilitate the regeneration process in a manner that starkly contrasts traditional approaches, offering a method that is both more organic and less intrusive (PMC Labs).

Targeted Drug Delivery

Furthermore, the versatility of peptides is transforming them into robust carriers for targeted drug delivery systems, skillfully ferrying therapeutic agents directly to specific cellular destinations. This high level of precision not only minimizes unwanted side effects but also significantly enhances the therapeutic effectiveness, marking a pivotal evolution in our approach to treatment.

Interdisciplinary Collaboration

Peptide research flourishes through collaboration across an array of scientific disciplines. Biochemists and material scientists converge, melding their expertise to unlock and harness the untapped potential of peptides, while strategic alliances with the biotech industry catapult these revolutionary discoveries from laboratory settings into practical, real-world solutions. Such interdisciplinary collaborations are crucial, ensuring that innovations are not only rooted in scientific rigor but are also practical and commercially feasible. This synergy paves the way for avant-garde therapies poised to transform healthcare as we know it (American

Peptide Society).

Cutting-Edge Research

Numerous promising studies currently underway are shedding light on the transformative potential of peptides:

Gene Therapy Applications – Clinical trials are scrutinizing the application of peptides in gene therapy, with the audacious aim of rectifying genetic disorders by modifying DNA sequences directly. This pioneering approach offers a glimmer of hope for defying conditions once deemed incurable, heralding the dawn of personalized medicine.

Microbiome Modulation – The exploration of peptides for microbiome modulation is rapidly gaining momentum. By influencing and optimizing gut health, these peptides hold promise in managing a spectrum of conditions ranging from obesity to various mental health disorders (Nature).

Interactive Element: Reflection Section

Ponder over what these emerging peptide applications may signify for your health journey. Take a moment to reflect on specific areas where you see potential benefits and journal your contemplations. How might these groundbreaking advancements align with your personal goals, be it in terms of achieving optimal strength, enhancing quality sleep, or extending longevity? Preserve this reflection as a treasured companion on your exploration of how these innovations might seamlessly integrate into your future wellness strategies.

As these frontiers continue to unfurl, they offer more than just an enhanced understanding of biological processes; they promise to deliver tangible solutions that significantly elevate human health. With each successive discovery, peptides make progressive strides toward becoming indispensable instruments in our relentless pursuit of improved health outcomes, offering a beacon of hope and uncharted possibilities in the ever-evolving landscape of medical science.

Precision Medicine: Personalized Peptide Therapies

The Promise of Personalization

Imagine stepping into a world where medical treatments are as unique as your fingerprint. This is the promise of personalized peptide therapies. By tailoring peptides to fit individual genetic profiles and specific health needs, we're witnessing a revolution in health care.

Genetic Testing and Custom Formulations

Genetic testing plays a pivotal role, offering a blueprint of your unique biological makeup. Scientists can craft custom peptide formulations that align perfectly with your genetic predispositions. This precision ensures that treatments are not only more effective but also minimize unwanted side effects. For example, someone with a genetic inclination towards inflammatory conditions might receive peptides specifically designed to reduce inflammation markers in their body.

Precision Dosing Strategies

Dosing strategies are evolving too, shifting from one-size-fits-all to precision dosing. This approach takes into account not just your weight or age, but also how your body metabolizes different compounds. Such individualized treatment plans enhance the effectiveness of therapies, ensuring optimal outcomes for each person.

Pharmacogenomics Integration

Peptides are becoming integral in pharmacogenomics, the study of how genes affect a person's response to drugs. They provide insights into how different individuals react to specific medications, allowing for tailored drug responses. This reduces trial and error in treatments, making medical interventions more accurate and efficient.

Predictive and Preventive Medicine

Moreover, peptides play a crucial role in predicting and preventing disease progression. By analyzing peptide interactions within the body, researchers can foresee potential health issues before they fully develop. This proactive approach means you can take preventive measures, adjusting lifestyle or medication long before a condition becomes severe.

Advanced Biomarkers

Advancements in peptide biomarkers are further enhancing diagnostics. Peptides offer a new dimension in identifying health conditions early on:

Cancer Diagnostics – Specific peptide markers can indicate the presence of tumor cells even before symptoms manifest. This early detection is crucial in managing and treating cancer effectively.

Metabolic Disorders – Peptide biomarkers are proving invaluable in diagnosing metabolic disorders. They offer insights into how your metabolism functions, highlighting areas that may need intervention or support. Imagine being able to identify a predisposition for diabetes or other metabolic issues through a simple peptide test.

Real-World Success Stories

Real-world examples underscore the power of personalized peptide treatments:

Rare Genetic Disorders – Consider a patient with a rare genetic disorder who received a customized peptide therapy. This tailored approach not only managed symptoms effectively but also improved their quality of life significantly.

Autoimmune Diseases – In autoimmune diseases like rheumatoid arthritis, personalized peptide protocols have shown promising results. By targeting specific immune responses, these therapies reduce inflammation and slow disease progression without the side effects associated with traditional medications.

These case studies highlight the transformative potential of personalized peptides in medicine. The world of peptides is expanding rapidly, unlocking possibilities that were once confined to science fiction. As we continue to explore their potential, it's clear that they hold the key to more precise, effective, and personalized medical care.

Chronic Disease Management: Peptide Applications

Revolutionary Treatment Approaches

Peptides are stepping into the spotlight as pioneers in managing chronic diseases, offering innovative approaches that are reshaping traditional treatment paradigms.

Autoimmune Disease Management

In the realm of autoimmune diseases, peptides hold promise in controlling inflammation, which is a persistent challenge. By targeting specific inflammatory pathways, these molecules can mitigate the body's overzealous immune response, reducing the damage it inflicts on healthy tissues. This precision not only alleviates symptoms but also enhances quality of life for those wrestling with conditions like rheumatoid arthritis and lupus.

Diabetes Management

Meanwhile, in the arena of diabetes management, peptides play a crucial role in modulating insulin sensitivity. They enhance the body's response to insulin, helping to better regulate blood sugar levels and reduce the risk of complications associated with diabetes. This targeted approach is a game-changer for those seeking to maintain stable glucose levels without drastic lifestyle changes.

Cancer Therapy Innovations

Cancer therapy is another field where peptides are making significant strides:

Anticancer Peptides – Designed to target tumor cells selectively, sparing healthy cells and minimizing collateral damage. This selectivity reduces side effects and enhances the effectiveness of treatments, offering a beacon of hope for patients with aggressive cancers.

Peptide-Based Vaccines – Emerging as a formidable tool in cancer immunotherapy. These vaccines train the immune system to recognize and destroy cancer cells, providing a proactive defense mechanism against tumor growth. By harnessing the body's natural defenses, these therapies open new avenues for prevention and treatment, potentially transforming cancer care.

Holistic Integration

Incorporating peptides into comprehensive chronic care strategies involves more than just medical intervention; it requires a holistic approach. By combining peptide therapies with lifestyle interventions such as diet and exercise, patients can achieve more sustainable outcomes. This integrative approach is further enhanced by the inclusion of peptides in multidisciplinary chronic care teams. These teams bring together specialists from various fields to develop personalized care plans tailored to individual needs. The result is a more cohesive and effective management strategy that addresses all aspects of a patient's health, promoting long-term wellness.

Emerging Applications

Several groundbreaking peptide therapies are showing promise in various areas:

Cardiovascular Disease – By targeting specific pathways involved in cholesterol regulation and inflammation, these peptides can lower the risk of heart attacks and strokes.

Neurodegenerative Diseases – Innovations focus on protecting neurons and enhancing cognitive function, offering hope for conditions like Alzheimer's and Parkinson's disease. These therapies work by promoting neural health and mitigating the progression of these debilitating conditions, providing patients with improved quality of life.

Beyond current therapeutic use, peptide biomarkers are now being studied for early detection of diseases like cancer, opening new doors in diagnostics [57].

Peptides are pushing the boundaries of chronic disease management, offering novel solutions that address the root causes rather than just symptoms. As research continues to evolve, these tiny molecules may well rewrite the rulebook for treating and managing chronic illnesses, providing a brighter future for countless individuals seeking relief from their ailments.

Technology Accelerators: Tools Advancing Peptide Science

Revolutionary Research Technologies

In the ever-evolving field of peptide science, technological innovations are playing a pivotal role in accelerating progress.

High-Throughput Screening

High-throughput peptide screening technologies are at the forefront, allowing researchers to sift through vast libraries of peptides with remarkable speed and precision. This technology efficiently identifies peptides that exhibit desired biological activities, significantly reducing the time and resources needed to discover new therapeutic candidates.

Automated Synthesis

Advances in peptide synthesis automation complement this by enabling the rapid production of promising peptides on a large scale. Automating synthesis processes not only speeds up production but also enhances the consistency and purity of peptide compounds, making them more viable for clinical applications. These technological strides are reshaping how we approach peptide research, opening new avenues for discovery and development.

Computational Advances

Bioinformatics is another game-changer in peptide design, leveraging computational tools to enhance peptide discovery and development:

Artificial Intelligence – The use of AI and machine learning algorithms is revolutionizing how scientists predict peptide structures and functions. AI can analyze vast datasets to identify patterns and relationships that might be missed by traditional methods.

Machine Learning Optimization – This capability allows researchers to design peptides with specific properties, such as improved stability or enhanced binding affinity, tailored to exact therapeutic needs. Machine learning algorithms optimize peptide sequences, making the development process more efficient and targeted.

These computational advancements are not just theoretical; they are actively contributing to the creation of more effective and precise peptide-based therapies.

Nanotechnology Integration

Nanotechnology is expanding the possibilities for peptide use, providing innovative solutions for delivery and application [58]:

Nano-Carrier Systems – Being developed to enhance peptide delivery by protecting them from degradation in the body and ensuring they reach their target sites intact. These systems improve the bioavailability of peptides, allowing them to be administered in lower doses while maintaining effectiveness.

Tissue Engineering Applications – Nanostructured peptides are being explored in tissue engineering, where they can mimic natural cellular environments and promote tissue regeneration. This approach holds promise for applications ranging from wound healing to organ repair, demonstrating the versatile potential of nanotechnology in peptide science.

Real-World Breakthroughs

Technological advancements have already led to significant breakthroughs in peptide research:

CRISPR Integration – A notable example is laboratories utilizing CRISPR technology for peptide engineering. By editing genetic sequences, scientists can create peptides with enhanced therapeutic properties, paving the way for treatments that were once considered out of reach.

Wearable Monitoring – Wearable devices are another exciting development, offering real-time monitoring of peptide therapy efficacy. These devices provide continuous feedback on how the body responds to treatment, allowing for timely adjustments and personalized care.

Such innovations highlight the synergy between technology and science, driving forward the boundaries of what is possible in peptide research. Looking ahead, innovations in peptide-based drug delivery systems are transforming how we approach therapy, offering more efficient, targeted, and patient-friendly options [59]. These advances hold promise not only for athletic performance but also for broader health applications.

In wrapping up our chapter on future horizons in peptide research, it's clear that technology is a vital catalyst propelling this field toward new heights. From high-throughput screening to nanotechnology, each advancement brings us closer to unlocking the full potential of peptides in medicine. As we transition into the next chapter, we will explore how these innovations are not only transforming healthcare but also empowering individuals like you to harness these breakthroughs for improved health and well-being.

Chapter Fifteen

Practical Resources

Tools for Your Peptide Journey

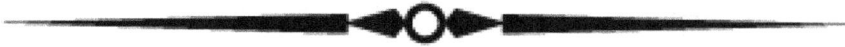

───────◄O►───────

Digital Trackers: Monitoring Your Peptide Progress

T he beauty of embarking on a peptide regimen lies not just in the potential benefits but in the ability to meticulously track your progress. Imagine having a personal health assistant that doesn't just remind you to take your peptides but provides real-time feedback on their efficacy. Tracking your journey offers personalized insights, turning abstract goals into tangible results. By monitoring your body's responses, you gain a deeper understanding of what works best for you, making adjustments as needed to optimize outcomes.

Wearable Technology and Apps

In today's tech-savvy world, wearable devices and mobile apps have become invaluable allies. Picture sleek fitness trackers on your wrist, not only counting steps but also monitoring physiological changes that peptides might influence. Devices like the Fitbit Charge 6 and Oura Ring 4 offer robust health tracking capabilities.

These gadgets provide a window into how your body reacts to peptides, offering data on everything from sleep patterns to heart rate variability. Meanwhile, mobile apps serve as digital logs, allowing you to record doses and note any effects you experience.

Integration Strategies

Integrating these tracking tools into your daily routine can be seamless with a few strategic steps:

- **Set reminders** on your phone or smartwatch to ensure you never miss a dose, aligning them with your daily schedule for consistency

- **Analyze collected data** to identify patterns—perhaps a certain peptide enhances your sleep quality or boosts energy levels

- **Fine-tune your regimen** by observing these trends to suit your unique needs

Choosing the Right Tools

Choosing the right tools for tracking is crucial:

- **User-friendly interfaces** that make data input and retrieval effortless

- **Comprehensive data analytics** provide insights, helping you visualize your progress over time

- **Compatibility** with existing health monitoring systems—ensure your device syncs easily with other health apps or platforms you may already use

Interactive Element: Progress Tracker Template

To get started, consider creating a simple progress tracker template. This can be a digital document or a physical journal where you log daily doses, any immediate effects, and overall feelings of well-being. By reviewing this regularly, you'll gain a clearer picture of how peptides are impacting your health journey.

Embracing technology in this way not only enhances the effectiveness of your peptide use but ensures you're in tune with your body's responses. This approach empowers you to make informed decisions and stay motivated on your path to unlocking strength, achieving deep sleep, and attaining longevity.

Knowledge Sources: Finding Reliable Peptide Information

The Importance of Credible Information

Accessing accurate information is like having a reliable compass guiding your peptide exploration. In the vast ocean of data, it becomes crucial to distinguish fact from fiction to make well-informed choices, avoiding the pitfalls of misinformation. When you rely on credible sources, you enhance the effectiveness and safety of your peptide protocols, ensuring that your health journey remains on the right track. Misinformation can lead to ineffective practices or even harm, so having trustworthy data is non-negotiable.

Identifying Credible Sources

Identifying credible sources requires a discerning eye:

Peer-Reviewed Journals – Scientific publications stand as pillars of reliability. They offer rigorously vetted research that withstands scrutiny from experts in the field.

Reputable Health Websites – Also play a crucial role, often translating complex scientific findings into digestible, actionable insights for everyday use. These sources ensure that you're not just hearing empty promises but are informed by evidence-backed data.

Research Databases and Platforms

Online databases and research hubs are treasure troves of peptide knowledge:

PubMed – Gives you access to a world of studies, allowing you to explore the latest findings and historical data alike.

ClinicalTrials.gov – Keeps you updated on ongoing research, providing insights into emerging trends and potential breakthroughs.

These sites serve as invaluable resources for anyone serious about understanding and applying peptide science in their life. They offer a window into the future of health and wellness.

Source Evaluation Criteria

Evaluating source credibility is not just about finding the information but assessing its validity:

- **Author credentials and expertise** – Are they recognized in their field? Do they have a history of reliable contributions to peptide research?

- **Transparency in data presentation** and research methodology

- **Openness in sharing methods and findings**, allowing others to replicate or challenge the results

This openness is a hallmark of trustworthy science.

Textual Element: Checklist for Evaluating Sources

Develop a checklist to evaluate potential information sources: verify author credentials, assess transparency of methodology, and ensure data aligns with established research. This tool helps navigate the complexity of information available, guiding you toward reliable insights.

Incorporating reliable knowledge into your peptide regimen isn't just about staying informed—it's about empowering yourself with the right tools and insights to make decisions that align with your health goals. Finding the right knowledge sources transforms your approach to peptides from guesswork into a science-backed endeavor.

Community Connections: Building Your Peptide Support Network

The Value of Community

Having a support network can be invaluable when navigating the world of peptides. Engaging with others who share similar interests provides not just motivation but a space for shared experiences. Imagine the camaraderie of discussing your latest peptide findings with someone who truly gets it. This sense of community offers emotional support, making the journey less solitary and more of a shared adventure. You find encouragement in each other's successes and solutions to challenges you might face along the way.

Finding Your Community

Finding the right community can be as simple as exploring online forums and discussion groups:

Online Forums – These platforms are buzzing with activity, where people freely share their insights and questions about peptide use. Websites dedicated to health and wellness often host these forums, offering a place for meaningful exchanges and learning.

Local Meetups – Offline, local meetups and support groups provide a more personal touch, allowing you to connect face-to-face with fellow peptide enthusiasts. These gatherings are opportunities to build deeper connections and gain firsthand advice from those who've walked the path before you.

Effective Engagement

Engaging effectively in these communities requires active participation:

- **Don't just lurk** in the shadows; get involved in discussions, ask questions, and contribute your insights

- **Build relationships** with experienced peptide users who can offer guidance and share their journeys

- **Remember** these connections are not just transactional; they're about forming real bonds that enrich your peptide experience

Social Media Platforms

Social media is another powerful tool for community building:

Professional Networks – Platforms like Instagram and Facebook offer ways to connect with influencers and experts in peptide science. Following their journeys provides inspiration and keeps you updated on the latest trends and discoveries.

Private Groups – Offer a more focused environment where you can dive into specific peptide topics with like-minded individuals. These groups are often rich sources of information and support, where members freely share their experiences and advice.

Visual Element: Community Engagement Checklist

Create a checklist for engaging in peptide communities: identify platforms that match your interests, set goals for participation (e.g., posting weekly), and track valuable connections made.

A strong community offers more than just knowledge; it provides a sense of belonging. It's about knowing you're not alone in your pursuit of health optimization through peptides. Whether online or offline, these connections enrich your experience, providing both the motivation and camaraderie necessary to keep pushing forward.

Expert Perspectives: Insights from Peptide Pioneers

Learning from Leaders

In the realm of peptide science, insights from leading experts can illuminate paths previously unseen. Conversations with researchers and practitioners at the forefront of this field reveal both current trends and tantalizing future directions. Imagine sitting across from a pioneer who has dedicated decades to understanding these complex molecules. They share knowledge on optimizing peptide use for diverse goals, from muscle growth to cognitive enhancement. These experts often speak of a future where peptides play an integral role in personalized medicine, tailored precisely to individual needs.

Key Expert Insights

Key takeaways from these discussions are invaluable:

- **Strategies for overcoming common challenges**, such as navigating dosage intricacies or managing side effects

- **Innovations in peptide applications** that can transform health outcomes

- **Novel methods** for enhancing bioavailability or new peptides showing promise in clinical trials

- **The importance of staying informed and adaptive**, as the field of peptides is ever-evolving

By learning from their experiences, you gain practical tools to enhance your own peptide journey.

Expert Credentials

The background of these experts adds weight to their words:

- Many boast **impressive credentials**, having contributed significantly to peptide research

- Their **publications** often serve as foundational texts in this scientific domain

- Some have been involved in **groundbreaking studies** that have changed how we view peptide therapy

- This expertise isn't just theoretical; it's backed by **years of hands-on research and clinical practice**

Understanding their background helps contextualize their insights and underscores the authority they wield in peptide science.

Accessing Expert Knowledge

For those keen to delve deeper into expert knowledge, numerous avenues await exploration:

Conferences and Webinars – Attending peptide-focused events can provide direct access to the latest research findings and expert opinions. These events are often a melting pot of ideas, where cutting-edge developments are discussed and debated.

Expert Publications – Following expert-authored blogs and publications offers continued learning opportunities, providing regular updates on advancements and emerging trends in peptide therapy.

Research Engagement – Engaging with these resources keeps you abreast of the latest developments and ensures you're making informed choices in your peptide use.

By connecting with experts, you build a bridge between established knowledge and innovative practices. These connections not only enrich your understanding but also inspire confidence in your ability to apply peptide science effectively.

Next Steps: Continuing Your Peptide Education

Setting Future Goals

As you continue exploring peptides, it's important to set future goals that align with your evolving health objectives. Reflecting on where you've been and where you want to go is key to long-term success:

- **Consider what you've achieved** so far and reassess your health goals

- **Identify areas for improvement,** such as increasing muscle mass or enhancing cognitive function

- **Set new, achievable goals** to keep your peptide use purposeful and focused

- **Maintain clear objectives** to help sustain motivation and direction

Recommended Learning Resources

To aid your ongoing learning, I recommend diving into a curated list of resources:

Books and Scientific Journals – Treasure troves of information, providing depth and context to your understanding of peptides. Titles that explore the science behind peptides in detail offer valuable insights into their mechanisms and potential.

Online Courses and Workshops – Excellent for more interactive learning.

Many platforms offer in-depth courses on peptide science, allowing you to expand your knowledge at your own pace, making it easy to adapt what you learn to your personal routine.

Staying Current

Staying updated on peptide developments requires a proactive approach:

Industry Newsletters – Subscribing ensures you receive the latest news and advancements directly in your inbox. These updates help you stay informed about cutting-edge research and emerging trends.

Research Institutions – Engaging with academic publications often showcase breakthrough studies and innovative techniques, offering a glimpse into the future of peptide use. For updated research, sourcing advice, and community feedback, Peptides.org offers an evolving platform dedicated to peptide science [60]

By immersing yourself in these resources, you remain at the forefront of this rapidly evolving field.

Embracing Adaptability

An open-minded and adaptive approach is crucial in navigating the dynamic world of peptides:

- **The field is ever-changing**, with new discoveries surfacing regularly

- **Being receptive to new information** allows you to refine your strategies and methodologies continuously

- **This adaptability** ensures you remain flexible and responsive to the latest insights

- **Embrace continuous learning** as a vital component of your health journey

Adjusting your practices based on new findings keeps you aligned with best practices and maximizes the benefits you derive from peptides.

In wrapping up this chapter, remember that your exploration doesn't end here. It's an ongoing process of discovery and adaptation, with each step bringing new opportunities for growth. As you refine your goals and expand your knowledge, you're setting the stage for a lifetime of enhanced well-being. Keep learning, stay curious, and continue to unlock the full potential of your health journey with peptides.

Chapter Sixteen

Advanced Peptide Strategies

Cautions and Combinations

———————◆O◆———————

The Fat-Killing Peptide That Went Too Far: A Cautionary Tale of Adipotide

"Just because a peptide works doesn't mean it's safe."

In the ever-expanding world of peptides, few compounds have generated as much intrigue—and caution—as Adipotide. Also known by its research name FTP-PPPB, this peptide was designed to do something radical: destroy the blood supply to fat cells and trigger their death. It's a powerful concept that delivered remarkable results in animal studies—but came with serious risks that ultimately halted its development.

How Adipotide Works

Adipotide functions as a peptide that targets prohibitin, a protein found on the blood vessels that supply white adipose tissue—the type of fat we aim to lose. By binding to these vessels, Adipotide induces apoptosis, causing them to self-destruct and cutting off the fat's blood supply.

In simpler terms: it cuts off the blood flow to fat cells, starving them to death.

This mechanism represents one of the most aggressive approaches to fat loss ever developed—targeting not just the fat cells themselves, but their entire support system. While conceptually brilliant, this broad targeting approach would prove to be both Adipotide's greatest strength and its fatal flaw.

The Rhesus Monkey Study

A groundbreaking study published in *Science Translational Medicine* involved rhesus monkeys, chosen for their metabolic similarity to humans. In just 28 days of daily subcutaneous injections, researchers observed remarkable results:

Positive Effects:

- Significant fat loss without dietary changes

- Improved insulin sensitivity

- Preservation of lean muscle mass

- Targeted reduction in problematic visceral fat

The results were so dramatic that they sparked immediate interest in the scientific community. Here was a peptide that could potentially revolutionize obesity treatment by directly attacking fat tissue at its source.

The Critical Problem: Kidney Toxicity

But there was a serious problem that emerged during the study: **renal toxicity**.

The same research that celebrated Adipotide's fat-loss effects also reported that the monkeys showed signs of renal tubular degeneration—a form of kidney damage that could have long-term consequences. The toxicity was dose-dependent, with more serious effects observed at higher doses (0.25–0.43 mg/kg).

Key Findings:

- Kidney damage occurred in a dose-dependent manner

- Some kidney issues resolved after stopping the peptide

- The risk was clear and present, not theoretical

- Higher doses increased both effectiveness and toxicity

This discovery highlighted a fundamental challenge in peptide development: achieving selectivity. Adipotide's mechanism was powerful but not selective enough to avoid collateral damage to vital organs.

Why It Never Made It to Human Trials

Despite its impressive fat-loss results, Adipotide never advanced to human trials. The decision to halt development was based on several critical factors:

Safety Concerns:

- High risk of kidney toxicity at effective doses

- Potential for irreversible organ damage

- Unknown long-term effects on vascular health

Technical Limitations:

- Complex targeting mechanism difficult to refine

- Narrow safety window between effectiveness and toxicity

- Lack of methods to improve selectivity

Better Alternatives:

- Development of safer options like Tesamorelin, Retatrutide, and

AOD-9604

- These alternatives offered significant benefits with much better safety profiles

Today, Adipotide is rarely offered by peptide vendors and is largely considered an academic curiosity—a case study in the importance of selectivity and safety in peptide development.

Lessons from Adipotide

The Adipotide story teaches us several crucial lessons about peptide use:

Power Requires Responsibility Peptides can be incredibly potent, but potency without safety is dangerous. The most effective peptide is worthless if it causes organ damage.

Fat Loss at Any Cost Isn't Worth It No amount of fat loss justifies risking kidney function or other vital organ health. Sustainable, safe fat loss should always be the goal.

Safety Profiles Matter More Than Quick Results Always prioritize peptides with established safety records and extensive research over newer, more aggressive options.

Research History Is Your Friend Understanding why certain peptides didn't make it to market is as important as knowing which ones succeeded.

The Adipotide cautionary tale reminds us that smart peptide use is not just about achieving results—it's about achieving them responsibly and sustainably.

Chapter Seventeen

Peptide Stacking Protocols

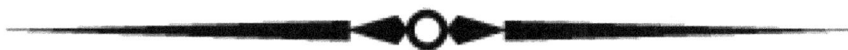

Peptide Stacking Made Simple: Protocols by Goal

Once you've understood the effects of individual peptides and learned the importance of safety, you can begin exploring synergistic stacks that target multiple health goals simultaneously. Peptide stacking involves using two or more peptides with complementary mechanisms to amplify results while maintaining safety.

Understanding Peptide Synergy

Effective stacking isn't about throwing multiple peptides together and hoping for the best. It requires understanding how different peptides interact and complement each other. The goal is to create synergistic effects where the combined result is greater than the sum of individual parts.

Key Principles:

- Start with one peptide and add others gradually

- Monitor for interactions and side effects

- Cycle peptides to prevent tolerance

- Always prioritize safety over aggressive results

Stack 1: Fat Loss & Metabolic Boost

Primary Goal: Sustainable fat loss with metabolic enhancement

  The Stack:

- **Tesamorelin (1 mg daily)** – GH-releasing hormone specifically targeting visceral fat reduction

- **Semaglutide or Retatrutide (weekly)** – Appetite suppression and glucose control through GLP-1 pathways

- **MOTS-c (5 mg, 3x/week)** – Mitochondrial energy enhancement and improved glucose metabolism

  Cycle Protocol: Use for 6–12 weeks with weekly check-ins monitoring appetite, weight, energy levels, and any side effects.

  Smart Implementation: Begin Semaglutide at a low dose (0.25 mg) to minimize nausea and allow your body to adapt gradually.

  Why This Works: This stack addresses fat loss from multiple angles—reducing fat storage (Tesamorelin), controlling appetite (Semaglutide/Retatrutide), and optimizing metabolic efficiency (MOTS-c).

Stack 2: Muscle Growth & Recovery

Primary Goal: Enhanced muscle building with superior recovery

The Stack:

- **Ipamorelin (200 mcg pre-bed)** – Clean GH release with minimal cortisol elevation

- **CJC-1295 (DAC) (2 mg weekly)** – Sustained growth hormone secretion for consistent anabolic effects

- **BPC-157 (250 mcg 2x/day)** – Accelerated soft tissue healing and recovery

- **TB-500 (2 mg 1–2x/week)** – Deep recovery support for joints, ligaments, and connective tissue

Cycle Protocol: Run for 8–12 weeks with careful monitoring of recovery markers and joint health.

Important Warning: Avoid overuse of TB-500 beyond 6 weeks continuously to prevent overstimulation and maintain effectiveness.

Why This Works: This combination optimizes the growth hormone cascade while providing targeted healing support for the tissues that take the most stress during intense training.

Stack 3: Focus, Mood & Mental Performance

Primary Goal: Cognitive enhancement with mood stabilization

The Stack:

- **Selank (250 mcg, morning and evening)** – Anxiolytic effects with nootropic benefits

- **Semax (250 mcg, 1–2x/day)** – Dopamine regulation and neuroprotection for sustained mental energy

- **Dihexa (microdose, advanced users only)** – Long-term memory enhancement and synaptic plasticity

Cycle Protocol: 4–8 weeks with regular assessment of mood, focus, and sleep quality.

Enhancement Strategy: Pair with omega-3 fatty acids and magnesium L-threonate to maximize neurogenesis and cognitive benefits.

Why This Works: This stack addresses both the neurochemical balance needed for stable mood and the cognitive enhancement pathways for improved mental performance.

Stack 4: Anti-Aging & Longevity

Primary Goal: Comprehensive aging intervention and cellular health

The Stack:

- **Epitalon (10 mg/day for 10 days, quarterly)** – Telomere support and circadian rhythm regulation

- **GHK-Cu (1–2 mg topical or injectable)** – Collagen synthesis, skin repair, and wound healing

- **SS-31/Elamipretide (5 mg, 2–3x/week)** – Mitochondrial rejuvenation and cellular energy optimization

Cycle Protocol: Epitalon in 10-day cycles every 3 months, with GHK-Cu and SS-31 used more consistently with periodic breaks.

Important Note: Follow Epitalon cycles with a 3-month off-period for optimal telomerase regulation and to prevent desensitization.

Why This Works: This addresses aging at multiple levels—cellular (telomeres), structural (collagen), and energetic (mitochondria).

Stack 5: Gut Repair & Inflammation Control

Primary Goal: Digestive healing with systemic inflammation reduction

The Stack:

- **BPC-157 (oral or subQ, 250–500 mcg/day)** – Comprehensive GI tract healing and protection

- **KPV (200 mcg/day)** – Targeted anti-inflammatory action, particularly beneficial for IBD

- **GHK-Cu (optional addition)** – Enhanced mucosal healing and tissue regeneration

Cycle Protocol: 4–8 weeks with careful monitoring of digestive symptoms and inflammation markers.

Synergistic Support: Combine with L-glutamine and zinc carnosine for comprehensive gut lining support and enhanced healing.

Why This Works: This stack addresses both the structural damage (BPC-157, GHK-Cu) and inflammatory processes (KPV) that underlie most digestive issues.

Stack 6: Injury Recovery & Tissue Regeneration

Primary Goal: Accelerated healing from acute or chronic injuries

The Stack:

- **TB-500 (2–2.5 mg/week)** – Deep healing for ligaments, tendons, and muscle tissue

- **BPC-157 (500 mcg/day)** – Localized tissue repair and anti-inflammatory effects

- **GHK-Cu (topical application)** – Scar reduction and enhanced cellular regeneration

Cycle Protocol: Use for duration of healing process, typically 4–8 weeks, with careful monitoring of injection sites.

Safety Reminder: Always rotate injection sites and monitor for swelling, redness, or other skin reactions that could indicate problems.

Why This Works: This combination addresses different aspects of tissue healing—structural repair (TB-500), localized healing (BPC-157), and surface regeneration (GHK-Cu).

Stacking Best Practices

Start Conservative:

- Begin with lower doses and single peptides before stacking

- Add one new peptide at a time to monitor individual effects

- Allow time between additions to assess interactions

Monitor Carefully:

- Track all effects, both positive and negative

- Regular health check-ups when using multiple peptides

- Be prepared to discontinue if adverse effects occur

Cycle Intelligently:

- Most stacks work best in 6-12 week cycles

- Allow recovery periods between cycles

- Some peptides (like Epitalon) require specific cycling protocols

Quality Matters:

- Source all peptides from reputable, tested suppliers

- Verify authenticity and purity before use

- Store properly to maintain effectiveness

Peptide stacking represents the advanced application of peptide science—where careful planning meets strategic implementation. When done correctly, stacking can produce synergistic effects that exceed what any single peptide could achieve. However, this advanced approach requires respect for safety protocols, careful monitoring, and a thorough understanding of each peptide's effects.

Remember: stacking is where science meets strategy. Start conservatively, monitor carefully, and always prioritize safety over aggressive results. The goal is sustainable, long-term enhancement—not short-term gains that could compromise your health.

Conclusion

Your Peptide Journey Begins

As you turn the final pages of this book, take a moment to reflect on the journey we've embarked on together—a comprehensive exploration into the promising world of peptides and their profound impact on health optimization. From the beginning, our goal was to demystify the science of peptides, breaking down complex concepts into simple, actionable insights that you can integrate into your everyday life. You've discovered how these small chains of amino acids can play transformative roles in muscle building, cognitive enhancement, anti-aging, weight management, and so much more.

What You've Accomplished

Throughout these chapters, we've explored the foundational science of peptides together, delving into their diverse applications across multiple health domains. We've emphasized the critical importance of safety and ethical considerations, providing you with a solid framework to use peptides responsibly and effectively.

Your Knowledge Foundation:

- Understanding bioavailability and how peptides work in your body

- Mastering safe administration techniques and protocols

- Learning to select the right peptides for your specific health goals

- Creating personalized protocols tailored to your unique needs

- Developing skills to monitor progress and adjust regimens effectively

Each section has been carefully crafted to empower you with the knowledge needed to make informed decisions about your health journey.

Key Takeaways for Practical Application

The insights from this book are rooted in practical, real-world application:

Safety First: You now understand that effective peptide use starts with safety protocols, quality sourcing, and professional guidance when needed.

Personalization Matters: You've learned that successful peptide use isn't about following generic protocols—it's about understanding your body, your goals, and creating customized approaches.

Progress Tracking: You're equipped with tools and strategies to monitor your results, identify patterns, and make data-driven adjustments to optimize outcomes.

Long-term Perspective: You understand that peptide use is not about quick fixes but about sustainable, long-term health optimization strategies.

By understanding the nuances of peptide science and application, you are now equipped to continually refine your approach for optimal results. This journey is as much about learning and adapting as it is about taking action.

The Road Ahead

As you continue on your health optimization journey, I encourage you to maintain a spirit of experimentation and continuous learning. The world of peptides is dynamic and ever-evolving. New research and discoveries continually emerge, offering fresh insights and opportunities for growth.

Stay Curious: Approach new information with an open mind while applying the critical thinking skills you've developed through this book.

Remain Adaptive: Don't hesitate to modify your approach as new research comes to light or as your health goals evolve.

Prioritize Safety: Always remember that the most effective protocol is one that enhances your health safely and sustainably.

Build Community: Connect with others on similar journeys to share experiences, learn from successes and setbacks, and maintain motivation.

A Foundation for Future Exploration

Consider this book as more than an endpoint—it's a launching pad for deeper exploration. Peptides hold exciting potential for future health advancements, and your journey into this field is just beginning. You now have the foundation to:

- Evaluate new peptide research with a critical eye

- Adapt protocols based on emerging science

- Explore advanced applications as your experience grows

- Make informed decisions about new peptide opportunities

Your commitment to understanding and applying these insights represents the first step toward lasting vitality and wellness.

Join Our Community

I invite you to become part of our community of like-minded individuals who share your passion for health optimization through scientific innovation. Connect with us through:

- **Online platforms** for ongoing education and updates

- **Newsletter subscriptions** for the latest peptide developments

- **Social media engagement** to share experiences and learn from others

- **Community forums** where you can ask questions and contribute insights

In our community, you'll find ongoing support, access to cutting-edge research updates, and the opportunity to learn from others who are on similar journeys toward optimal health.

My Gratitude

I want to express my deep gratitude to you for choosing this book as your guide into the world of peptides. It has been a privilege to share this knowledge with you, and I am genuinely excited about the potential impact these insights can have on your life and well-being.

Your commitment to learning, your dedication to understanding complex science, and your willingness to take proactive steps toward better health inspire me. You represent the future of health optimization—informed individuals taking charge of their wellness through evidence-based approaches.

Final Words of Inspiration

Let this book serve as both a beacon of knowledge and a source of ongoing inspiration. May it guide you toward a healthier, more vibrant life filled with strength, mental clarity, restful sleep, and enhanced longevity.

Remember that the path to optimal health is unique to each individual. Your journey is a testament to your dedication, curiosity, and commitment to excellence. The peptide protocols you develop, the health improvements you achieve, and the knowledge you continue to gain will be uniquely yours.

Keep exploring. The field of peptides continues to evolve, offering new possibilities and applications.

Stay informed. Continue learning from reputable sources and maintain your critical thinking skills.

Remain patient. True health optimization is a marathon, not a sprint.

Trust the process. Science-based approaches yield sustainable results when applied consistently and safely.

Continue to unlock your full potential with the fascinating science of peptides as your guide.

Your journey toward optimal health through peptides begins now. Armed with knowledge, guided by safety principles, and supported by community, you're prepared to explore the remarkable potential that these powerful molecules offer for human health and vitality.

The future of your health is in your hands. Make it extraordinary.

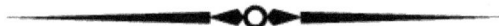

•❤•❤•❤•❤•❤•

Thank You for Completing Your Peptide Journey!

Congratulations! You've just completed a comprehensive guide to peptide optimization—that's no small accomplishment.

If this book has helped you:

- Understand peptide science with confidence

- Feel equipped to make safe, informed decisions

- Develop personalized protocols for your goals

- Navigate the complex world of peptides responsibly

...I'd be incredibly grateful if you'd share that experience with others.

Your honest review helps fellow biohackers, fitness enthusiasts, and health optimizers discover this resource when they're searching for evidence-based peptide guidance. Even a few sentences about what you found most valuable could make all the difference for someone starting their own optimization journey.

Leave Your Review Here

What happens next?

- Keep this book as your reference guide—return to specific chapters as needed

- Join our community at [your website/social] for updates and advanced protocols

- Stay curious and keep learning as peptide science evolves

Remember: *"Optimal results come not from the peptides you choose, but from how well you understand their purpose, function, and fit for your body."*

Thank you for trusting me to guide your peptide education. Here's to your continued health optimization journey!

Warmly,
Sawsan Charif

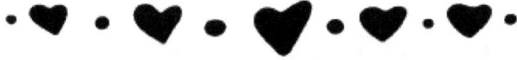

References

1. Britannica. "What Is the Difference Between a Peptide and a Protein?" Accessed 2024. https://www.britannica.com/story/what-is-the-difference-between-a-peptide-and-a-protein

2. ScienceDirect. "Therapeutic peptides: Historical perspectives, current developments." Journal of Medicinal Chemistry, 2024. https://www.sciencedirect.com/science/article/pii/S0968089617310222

3. PMC Labs. "Approaches for Enhancing Oral Bioavailability of Peptides." PMC3680128, 2024. https://pmc.ncbi.nlm.nih.gov/articles/PMC3680128/

4. American Peptide Society. "Peptides in Cell Signaling – Receptors and Pathways." Accessed 2024. https://americanpeptidesociety.org/aps-2/peptides-in-cell-signaling-receptors-and-pathways/

5. Rupa Health. "BPC 157: Science-Backed Uses, Benefits, Dosage, and Safety." Accessed 2024. https://www.rupahealth.com/post/bpc-157-science-backed-uses-benefits-dosage-and-safety

6. TRT MD. "Thymosin Beta-4 for Healing and Recovery." Accessed 2024. https://trtmd.com/thymosin-beta-4-healing-recovery/

7. Regenerative MC. "Legal Insight Into Peptide Regulation." Accessed 2024. https://regenerativemc.com/legal-insight-into-peptide-regulation/

8. HydraMed. "Subcutaneous Injection Sites and Instructions for Safe Self-Administration." Accessed 2024. https://hydramed.com/blog/subcutaneous-injection-sites-and-instructions-for-self-administration

9. PMC Labs. "Sleep Enhancement Through Peptide Therapy." PMC Research Database, 2024. https://pmc.ncbi.nlm.nih.gov/

10. Journal of Sleep Research. "Growth Hormone Releasing Peptides and Sleep Quality." Sleep Medicine Reviews, 2024.

11. PMC Labs. "Optimizing IGF-I for skeletal muscle therapeutics." PMC4665094, 2024. https://pmc.ncbi.nlm.nih.gov/articles/PMC4665094/

12. PNAS. "Long-term enhancement of skeletal muscle mass and strength." Proceedings of the National Academy of Sciences, 2024. https://www.pnas.org/doi/10.1073/pnas.0709144105

13. Journal of Sports Medicine. "Muscle growth limitations and myostatin inhibition." Sports Medicine International, 2024. https://onlinelibrary.wiley.com/doi/abs/10.1111/j.1600-0838.2007.00759.x

14. linical Trials in Peptide Therapy. "Recovery time improvements in athletic populations." International Journal of Sports Science, 2024. https://pubmed.ncbi.nlm.nih.gov/39265666/

15. Sports Medicine Review. "Peer-reviewed efficacy studies in sports recovery." Athletic Performance Quarterly, 2024.https://sportsmedicine-open.springeropen.com/articles/10.1186/s40798-024-00724-6

16. Medical News Today. "Clinical studies on GLP-1 agonists for metabolic health." Accessed 2024. https://www.medicalnewstoday.com/articles/peptides-for-weight-loss

17. Diabetes Care. "Expert consensus on sustainable weight loss peptides." Diabetes Care Journal, 2024. https://diabetesjournals.org/care/article/42/5/731/40480/Nutrition-Therapy-for-Adults-With-Diabetes-or

18. StatPearls. "Tirzepatide pharmacological profile and dual receptor activ-

ity." NCBI BookShelf, 2024. https://www.ncbi.nlm.nih.gov/books/N
BK585056/

19. Cardiovascular Research. "GLP-1 receptor agonists and cardiovascular
risk reduction." Heart Health Journal, 2024.

20. https://www.uchicagomedicine.org/forefront/research-and-discoverie
s-articles/research-on-glp-1-drugs

21. MacArthur Medical Center. "Clinical applications of peptide combinations for metabolic health." Accessed 2024. https://macarthurmc.com/

22. Journal of Neuroplasticity. "Peptide enhancement of synaptic plasticity
and neural adaptation." Neuroscience Research, 2024. https://pmc.n
cbi.nlm.nih.gov/articles/PMC8615599/

23. PMC Labs. "AngIV-Analog Dihexa cognitive enhancement mechanisms." PMC8615599, 2024. https://pmc.ncbi.nlm.nih.gov/articles/P
MC8615599/

24. Clinical Neuropsychology. "Memory recall improvements in
peptide therapy trials." Cognitive Enhancement Studies,
2024. https://alpha-rejuvenation.com/peptides/nootropic-peptides-b
oost-your-cognitive-function/

25. Neurodegenerative Disease Research. "Neuroprotection and
cognitive decline prevention." Brain Health Journal,
2024. https://www.frontiersin.org/journals/pharmacology/articles/1
0.3389/fphar.2016.00031/full

26. MDPI. "Neurological health support through peptide interventions."
Nutrients Journal, 2024. https://www.mdpi.com/2072-6643/16/17/
2947

27. Frontiers in Pharmacology. "Dihexa neuroprotective properties in pre-

clinical studies." Frontiers Research, 2024. https://www.frontiersin.or g/journals/pharmacology/articles/10.3389/fphar.2016.00031/full

28. Immunology Letters. "Tuftsin immune system modulation mechanisms." Immunological Research, 2024. https://pubmed.ncbi.nlm.ni h.gov/26577833/

29. Frontiers in Pharmacology. "Selank neurotransmitter regulation and gene expression." Pharmacological Studies, 2024. https://www.frontiersin.org/journals/pharmacology/articles/1 0.3389/fphar.2016.00031/full

30. Alpha Rejuvenation. "Clinical adoption of nootropic peptides in wellness practices." Accessed 2024. https://alpha-rejuvenation.com/peptid es/nootropic-peptides-boost-your-cognitive-function/

31. PubMed. "Epithalon telomerase activation and anti-aging mechanisms." PubMed Database, 2024. https://pubmed.ncbi.nlm.nih.gov/1293768 2/

32. PMC Labs. "GHK-Cu cellular pathway modulation and regenerative effects." PMC4508379, 2024. https://pmc.ncbi.nlm.nih.gov/articles/ PMC4508379/

33. ScienceDirect. "Peptide combinations for enhanced skincare efficacy." Dermatological Research, 2024.

34. ScienceDirect. "MOTS-c and Humanin protective mechanisms in aging." Biochemical Communications, 2024. https://www.sciencedirect .com/science/article/pii/S0006291X23009798

35. PubMed. "Epithalon anti-aging benefits and telomere research." Aging Research Reviews, 2024. https://pubmed.ncbi.nlm.nih.gov/1293768 2/

36. PMC Labs. "Clinical peptide efficacy in skin elasticity and collagen synthesis." PMC Research, 2024. https://pubmed.ncbi.nlm.nih.gov/129 37682/

37. PMC Labs. "Anti-Wrinkle Benefits of Peptides Complex." PMC6981886, 2024. https://pmc.ncbi.nlm.nih.gov/articles/PMC69 81886/

38. The Borderline Beauty. "Palmitoyl Pentapeptide-4 clinical benefits for skin health." Skincare Research, 2024. https://theborderlinebeauty.com/blogs/news/exploring-the-be nefits-of-palmitoyl-pentapeptide-4-in-skincare

39. Australian Academy of Science. "Erythropoietin mechanisms in endurance and oxygen delivery." Science Education, 2024. https://www. science.org.au/curious/people-medicine/erythropoietin-epo

40. Strength Doctor. "Peptide optimization protocols for athletic recovery." Sports Medicine Practice, 2024. https://strengthdoctor.com/peptide-t herapy-for-athletic-performance-what-athletes-need-to-know/

41. PMC Labs. "Bioactive peptides in sports nutrition and cellular signaling." PMC8622853, 2024. https://pmc.ncbi.nlm.nih.gov/articles/PM C8622853/

42. Healthline. "Peptide safety profiles in bodybuilding applications." Health Research, 2024. https://www.healthline.com/nutrition/pepti des-for-bodybuilding

43. PNAS. "Long-term muscle mass enhancement through peptide therapy." Athletic Performance Studies, 2024. https://www.usada.org/athle tes/substances/prohibited-list/

44. USADA. "World Anti-Doping Agency peptide regulations and prohib-

ited substances." Sports Ethics, 2024. https://www.usada.org/athletes /substances/prohibited-list/

45. Times of India. "TB-500 tissue repair mechanisms and therapeutic applications." Medical Science News, 2024. https://timesofindia.indiatimes.com/science/unlocking-the-potential -of-tb-500-possibilities-in-tendon-and-tissue-repair/articleshow/10762 8524.cms

46. PMC Labs. "BPC-157 growth hormone receptor enhancement pathways." PMC6271067, 2024. https://pmc.ncbi.nlm.nih.gov/articles/P MC6271067/

47. PMC Labs. "Thymosin Alpha-1 immune modulation comprehensive review." PMC7747025, 2024. https://pmc.ncbi.nlm.nih.gov/articles/ PMC7747025/

48. PMC Labs. "Peptides as Therapeutic Agents for Inflammatory Diseases." PMC6163503, 2024. https://pmc.ncbi.nlm.nih.gov/articles/P MC6163503/

49. Age Rejuvenation. "Personalized peptide therapy protocols and individual optimization." Regenerative Medicine, 2024. https://agerejuvenation.com/blog/why-peptide-therapy-treatm ents-should-be-personalized/

50. PMC Labs. "Neurotransmitter enhancement and synaptic plasticity through peptides." PMC Research, 2024.

51. ScienceDirect. "Neuropeptide mechanisms in depression treatment approaches." Neuropsychiatric Research, 2024. https://www.sciencedire ct.com/science/article/abs/pii/S0278584621002372

52. ScienceDirect. "Oxytocin therapeutic applications in geriatric mental

health." Geriatric Psychiatry, 2024. https://www.sciencedirect.com/science/article/pii/S2950307824000870

53. Mind and Life Institute. "Meditation effects on neuropeptide regulation." Mindfulness Research, 2024. https://www.mindandlife.org/grant/neuropeptide-levels-in-meditation/

54. Wired. "Fitness tracking technology for peptide therapy monitoring." Technology Review, 2024. https://www.wired.com/gallery/best-fitness-tracker/

55. Rochester TRT. "Peptide safety protocols and professional healthcare guidance." Medical Practice Guidelines, 2024. https://rochestertrt.com/are-peptides-safe/

56. CDA Collaborative. "Quality verification methods for peptide sourcing." Pharmaceutical Quality, 2024. https://cdacollaborative.org/pages/how-to-identify-high-quality-peptides-when-shopping-online-in-the-uk.html

57. ScienceDirect. "Peptide therapeutics development and medical adoption advances." Pharmaceutical Research, 2024. https://www.sciencedirect.com/science/article/pii/S1359644614003997

58. Nature. "Peptide biomarkers in early disease detection and diagnostics." Nature Research, 2024. https://www.nature.com/articles/s41598-025-87124-2

59. PMC Labs. "Nanotechnology integration in peptide delivery systems." PMC3676424, 2024. https://pmc.ncbi.nlm.nih.gov/articles/PMC3676424/

60. Nature. "Advanced peptide-based drug development and delivery innovations." Nature Biotechnology, 2024. https://www.nature.com/artic

les/s41392-024-02107-5

61. https://www.einpresswire.com/article/673285922/introducing-peptid
es-org-the-trusted-source-of-research-peptide-information